RENAL PHYSIOLOGY

NOTICE

Medicine is an ever-changing science. As new research and clinical experience broaden our knowledge, changes in treatment and drug therapy are required.

The author and the publisher of this work have checked with sources believed to be reliable in their efforts to provide information that is complete and generally in accord with the standards accepted at the time of publication. However, in view of the possibility of human error or changes in medical sciences, neither the author nor the publisher nor any other party who has been involved in the preparation or publication of this work warrants that the information contained herein is in every respect accurate or complete. Readers are encouraged to confirm the information contained herein with other sources. For example and in particular, readers are advised to check the product information sheet included in the package of each drug they plan to administer to be certain that the information contained in this book is accurate and that changes have not been made in the recommended dose or in the contraindications for administration. This recommendation is of particular importance in connection with new or infrequently used drugs.

5th EDITION

RENAL PHYSIOLOGY

Arthur J. Vander, M.D.
Professor Emeritus of Physiology
University of Michigan

McGraw-Hill, Inc.
HEALTH PROFESSIONS DIVISION

New York · St. Louis · San Francisco · Auckland · Bogotá · Caracas
Lisbon · London · Madrid · Mexico City · Milan · Montreal
New Delhi · San Juan · Singapore · Sydney · Tokyo · Toronto

RENAL PHYSIOLOGY

4 5 6 7 8 9 0 DOC DOC 9 8

This book was set in Times Roman by Northeastern Graphic Services, Inc.;
the editors were William Lamsback and Mariapaz Ramos-Englis; the
production supervisor was Richard C. Ruzycka. The text and cover were designed
by Marsha Cohen, Parallelogram. This project was managed by Hockett Editorial Service.

This book is printed on acid-free paper.

ISBN 0-07-067009-9

Library of Congress Catalog-in-Publication Data

Vander, Arthur J., date–
    Renal physiology / Arthur J. Vander. — 5 ed.
        p.   cm.
    Includes bibliographical references and index.
    ISBN 0-07-067009-9 (alk. paper)
    1. Kidneys—Physiology.   I. Title.
    [DNLM: 1. Kidney—physiology.   WJ 301 V229r   1995]
QP249.V36 1995
612.4′88—dc20
DNLM/DLC
for Library of Congress   94-27777

CONTENTS

5 RENAL HANDLING OF ORGANIC SUBSTANCES   79

6 BASIC RENAL PROCESSES FOR SODIUM, CHLORIDE, AND WATER   89

PREFACE

This book is my attempt to identify the essential core content of renal physiology appropriate for medical students and to present it in a way that permits the student to use the book as his or her primary learning resource. I have been gratified by the wide use the first four editions have achieved and the many letters I have received from medical students (and clinicians) who found they were, indeed, able to master its contents by independent study.

CHANGES IN THIS EDITION

My major goal in preparing this fifth edition has been to update the material completely but not to alter the level of coverage. Where appropriate, new topics have been added to the text or expanded, while the coverage of others has been completely redone because of changes in knowledge. A partial list of these topics follows (these relate only to the text proper; as described below, other new material, particularly on molecular mechanisms, has been added to the end-of-chapter notes):

Distribution and functions of type-A and type-B intercalated cells
New reference table of intrarenal chemical messengers (e.g., IGF-1, endothelin, nitric oxide)
Effects of the renal nerves and angiotensin II on renal hemodynamics
New reference table of vasoactive agents that act on the kidneys
Solvent drag
Transtubular potentials, their distribution and role in ion transport
Model of active organic anion secretion (PAH)
Overview of the regulation of membrane channels and transporters
Overview of tubular division of labor (proximal tubule as "mass transporter," etc.)
Comparison models of sodium and chloride transport in major tubular segments
Mechanism of active chloride transport in proximal tubule
Emphasis on nonreflex control of sodium reabsorption
Role of paracrine factors in sodium reabsorption

Determinants and role of renal interstitial hydraulic pressure
Pressure natriuresis
Atrial natriuretic factor
Effect of ADH on sodium reabsorption by cortical collecting duct
Effect of ADH on potassium secretion by cortical collecting duct
Role of H,K-ATPase in potassium reabsorption
Identities and distribution of the three types of hydrogen-ion trans-
    porters
Bicarbonate co- and countertransporters
Effects of angiotensin II and the renal nerves on hydrogen-ion
    secretion
Potassium depletion and ammonium synthesis
Molecular mechanisms of calcium reabsorption

In addition, several chapters have been reorganized: (1) A very small introductory section on basic renal processes (filtration, reabsorption, and secretion) now appears in Chapter 1. (2) The material on renal blood flow and glomerular filtration previously divided between Chapters 2 and 5 is now all in Chapter 2. (3) The material on basic mechanisms of reabsorption and secretion previously in Chapter 2 now forms a separate chapter (Chapter 4), which serves as an introduction to the remaining chapters of the book. Also, a summary table of all the reabsorptive and secretory processes carried out by each major tubular segment is found in new Appendix A, along with another summary table of the functions of the three cell types that constitute the collecting ducts.

Finally, much rewriting was done solely to increase clarity even though no updating was required. By cutting material no longer deemed essential I have managed to keep the size of the text proper unchanged. The expansion of the total book by a few pages is due entirely to an expansion of the end-of-chapter notes and the addition of new review and reference tables, which students have found to be very useful.

The illustration program has also undergone considerable revision. Fifteen new figures have been added, 15 eliminated, and 24 others significantly revised. Color has been added for the first time to enhance the educational value of the figures. Also, 12 new tables have been added, for I have found that these greatly aid in review or provide easy reference to material not to be memorized.

HOW TO USE THIS BOOK

As in previous editions, my selection of the core material is made explicit in a comprehensive list of behavioral objectives, which tell students specifically what I believe they should know and be able to do by the time they complete the book. Obviously, no two instructors would come up with exactly the same core material, but it is a simple matter for instructors to give students a supplementary list of objectives to be added or deleted. Of much greater importance is the fact that the behavioral objectives are explicitly defined so that any such differences are easily determined. This also makes the book quite usable for students in other health sciences, whose required core of information may differ from that of medical students.

In addition to the comprehensive objectives, I have included a large number of study questions with annotated answers. Unlike the lists of objectives, the study questions are neither systematic nor comprehensive in their coverage. Rather, they generally deal with areas I have found to be difficult for students.

I suggest that the student first go through a chapter purely with the goal of *understanding* what is in it, not striving to memorize any material at this time. Then go through it again, this time using the objectives to guide your learning. This is a very important point: By using the objectives, you will see that some material, particularly in the realms of quantitation and mechanisms, is presented for interest in order to facilitate the learning of general principles, and for reference, but is not meant for memorization. You should treat each objective as though it were an essay question. Then you should answer the study questions (at the back of the book) for that chapter. Together, the objectives and study questions provide means for determining whether you have mastered the material and for identifying those specific areas that require more work. Also, an excellent way to review a chapter quickly is to go over all the figures (including their legends) and tables in the chapter, since a large fraction of the important material is summarized in them. (Keep in mind, however, that some of the figures and tables, as stated in the text, are included purely for reference.)

COMPLEXITY AND THE END-OF-CHAPTER NOTES

The question of how to handle the growing complexity of renal physiology in an introductory textbook is a particularly perplexing one. First, for many specific phenomena (for example, sodium reabsorption even within a single tubular segment, or the control of renin secretion) there is a multiplicity of processes and controls; to deal with this I have often used the qualifiers "major" or "most important" when describing those processes and controls I chose to include in the text. Second, there has been an incredible expansion in our knowledge of the molecular mechanisms that underlie many of the processes and controls. Third, many statements of "fact" in renal physiology still remain uncertain and/or controversial. Fourth, additional information (for example, mechanisms by which drugs likely to be developed may act) may be useful in the future but is not directly applicable to clinical medicine at present.

As in past editions, I continue to use "notes," which in this edition have been moved to the backs of chapters, to describe at least some of the material in these four categories (as well as additional information that is just plain interesting to me). Often the decision to put something in a note is simply arbitrary. After much soul-searching I decided to expand these notes mainly so as to make the book more useful to the interested student and to have the information available should any instructor feel that a particular fact belongs to the core material. (In other words, I have often put into a note material that I chose not to include in the text but that, for good reasons, other instructors might feel should be learned by their students.) **My advice to the great majority of students is to ignore the end-of-chapter notes completely** except, of course, in those cases where the instructor assigns it.

Another characteristic of this book, as of most introductory textbooks, is that it contains almost none of the original research upon which the core of presented knowledge rests. To ensure that any interested student can gain entry to this research base as well as pursue any subject in greater depth, I have included an extensive list of suggested readings at the back of the book. Almost all are recent review articles, and their bibliographies provide an entry into the original research literature.

APPENDICES

Because the last five chapters of this book are organized around individual substances (sodium, potassium, etc.) rather than individual tubular segments, information about these segments is distributed among several chapters. To permit the student to see it all in one place, Appendix A contains two tables that summarize all the reabsorptive and secretory processes described in the text, arranged by tubular segment; they offer, therefore, an excellent review and/or reference after completing the book. Appendix B summarizes in tabular form the mechanisms by which the most commonly used diuretic drugs act and, therefore, constitutes another review of certain transport processes.

RENAL PHYSIOLOGY

RENAL FUNCTIONS, ANATOMY, AND BASIC PROCESSES

Objectives

The student knows the functions of the kidneys:

1 Lists the functions, including the three hormones secreted
2 States the role of erythropoietin and the stimulus for its secretion
3 States the components of the renin-angiotensin system and their biochemical interrelations

The student defines important gross structures and knows their interrelationships: renal pelvis, calyxes, renal pyramids, renal medulla (inner and outer zones), renal cortex, papilla.

The student understands the interrelationships between the components of a nephron:

1 Defines nephron, renal corpuscle, glomerulus (glomerular capillaries), and tubule
2 Draws the relationship between glomerulus, Bowman's capsule, and the proximal tubule
3 States the three layers separating the lumen of the glomerular capillaries and Bowman's space; defines podocytes, foot processes, slits, and slit diaphragms
4 Defines glomerular mesangial cells and states their functions
5 Lists in order all the individual tubular segments; states the segments that make up the proximal tubule, Henle's loop, and the collecting-duct system; defines principal cells and intercalated cells

The student lists in order the vessels through which blood flows from renal artery to renal vein; contrasts the blood supply to the cortex and the medulla; defines vasa recta and vascular bundles.

The student describes, in general terms, the differences between superficial cortical, midcortical, and juxtamedullary nephrons.

The student defines juxtaglomerular apparatus and describes its three cell types; states the function of the granular cells.

The student describes the innervation of the nephron.

The student defines the basic renal processes:

1 Defines glomerular filtration, tubular reabsorption, and tubular secretion
2 Lists the questions to be asked about the renal handling of any substance
3 Defines renal metabolism of a substance and gives examples

The student describes how angiotensin II and the eicosanoids are produced within the kidneys and can function as intrarenal chemical messengers.

FUNCTIONS

The kidneys process blood by removing substances from it and, in a few cases, by adding substances to it. In so doing, they perform a variety of functions, as summarized in Table 1-1.

The major function is to regulate the volume, osmolarity, mineral composition, and acidity of the body by excreting water and inorganic electrolytes in amounts adequate to achieve total-body balance of these substances and maintain their normal concentrations in the extracellular fluid. Ions regulated in this way include sodium, potassium, chloride, calcium, magnesium, sulfate, phosphate, and hydrogen ion.[1] (The superscript number at the end of the last sentence denotes an end-of-chapter note; I suggest that if you have not already done so you read what I have said about these notes in the Preface.) The kidneys also take part in a similar homeostatic regulation of some organic nutrients.

A second renal (the adjective denoting kidney) function is the excretion of metabolic **waste products**, so termed because they serve no function. These

Table 1-1 Functions of the Kidneys

1 Regulation of water and inorganic-ion balance
2 Removal of metabolic waste products from the blood and their excretion in the urine
3 Removal of foreign chemicals from the blood and their excretion in the urine
4 Gluconeogenesis
5 Secretion of hormones
 a Renin
 b Erythropoietin
 c 1,25-dihydroxyvitamin D_3

include urea (from protein), uric acid (from nucleic acids), creatinine (from muscle creatine), the end products of hemoglobin breakdown (which give urine much of its color), the metabolites of various hormones, and many others.

A third renal function is the excretion, in the urine, of many foreign chemicals—drugs, pesticides, food additives, and so on—and their metabolites.

A fourth renal function is gluconeogenesis. During prolonged fasting, the kidneys synthesize glucose from amino acids and other precursors and release it into the blood. The kidneys are capable of supplying approximately 20 percent as much glucose as the liver at such times.

Finally, the kidneys act as endocrine glands, secreting at least three hormones; 1,25-dihydroxyvitamin D_3, erythropoietin, and renin.

1,25-dihydroxyvitamin D_3 is the active form of vitamin D; its synthesis by the kidneys and its role in calcium metabolism are described in Chapter 10.

Erythropoietin is a peptide hormone that is involved in the control of erythrocyte production by the bone marrow. Its major source is the kidneys, although the liver also secretes small amounts. The renal cells that secrete it are a particular group of cells in the interstitium. The stimulus for its secretion is a reduction in the partial pressure of oxygen in the kidneys, as occurs, for example, in anemia, arterial hypoxia, or inadequate renal blood flow.[2] Erythropoietin stimulates the bone marrow to increase its production of erythrocytes. Renal disease may result in diminished erythropoietin secretion, and the ensuing decrease in bone marrow activity is one important causal factor in the anemia of chronic renal disease.

Renin, a component of the **renin-angiotensin system**, is a proteolytic enzyme secreted by the kidneys, specifically by the granular cells of the juxtaglomerular apparatuses (see below). Once in the bloodstream, renin catalyzes the splitting of a decapeptide, **angiotensin I**, from a plasma protein known as **angiotensinogen**, which is produced mainly by the liver and is always present in the plasma in high concentration (Fig. 1-1). Under the influence of another enzyme, **angiotensin-converting enzyme**, the terminal two amino acids are then split from the relatively inactive angiotensin I to yield the highly active octapeptide **angiotensin II.** Some angiotensin-converting enzyme is present in plasma, but most is on the endothelial surface of blood vessels throughout the body, including the kidneys. The pulmonary capillaries are particularly rich in this enzyme, and so a large fraction of plasma angiotensin I is converted to angiotensin II as blood flows through the lungs. What is rate-limiting in the renin-angiotensin system? Because angiotensinogen and angiotensin-converting enzyme are normally present in high and relatively unchanging concentrations, the primary determinant of the rate of angiotensin II formation is the plasma concentration of renin. (The control of renin secretion will be described in Chapter 5.)[3]

It should be noted at this point that certain tissues and organs other than the kidneys (e.g., the brain, heart, and uterus) can also produce both renin (or renin isoforms) and angiotensinogen. Since, as noted earlier, angiotensin-converting enzyme is widespread on capillary endothelium, the result is that

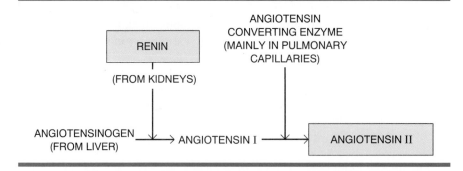

Fig. 1-1   Basic biochemistry of the renin-angiotensin system.

all the components required for generation of angiotensin II are contained locally in these particular tissues and organs. In other words, there are *completely local, nonrenal* renin-angiotensin systems; the angiotensin II produced by these systems acts locally as a paracrine agent. The roles of these nonrenal systems are the subject of much study but will, in general, not be discussed in this book. (See articles by Ganong; Baker et al.; and Lindpaintner and Ganten, in Suggested Readings.)

The many functions of angiotensin II will be described in subsequent chapters and are summarized for reference in Fig. 7-10. It is enough for now merely to state that the common denominators of most of them are to increase arterial blood pressure and cause sodium retention in the body.

ANATOMY OF THE KIDNEYS AND URINARY SYSTEM

The kidneys are paired organs that lie outside the peritoneal cavity in the posterior abdominal wall, one on each side of the vertebral column. The medial border of the kidney is indented by a deep fissure (called the hilum) through which pass the renal vessels and nerves and in which lies the **renal pelvis**, the funnel-shaped continuation of the upper end of the ureter (Fig. 1-2). The outer convex border of the renal pelvis is divided into major *calyxes,* each of which subdivides into several minor calyxes. Each of the latter is cupped around the projecting apex of a cone-shaped mass of tissue, a *renal pyramid.*

When the kidney is bisected from top to bottom it can be seen to be divided into two major regions: an inner **renal medulla** and an outer **renal cortex.** The medulla is made up of a number of renal pyramids, the apexes of which, as stated in the previous paragraph, project into the minor calyxes. Each apical tip is called a **papilla.** Each pyramid of the medulla, topped by a region of renal cortex, forms a single lobe.

Upon closer gross examination, additional features can be discerned: (1) The cortex has a highly granular appearance, absent in the medulla; and (2) each medullary pyramid is divisible into an **outer zone** (adjacent to the cortex)

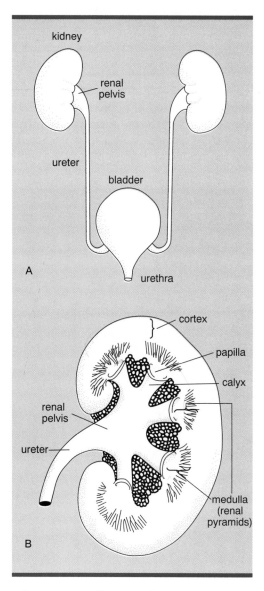

Fig. 1-2 (A) The urinary system. The urine formed by a kidney collects in the renal pelvis and then flows through the ureter into the bladder, from which it is eliminated via the urethra. (B) Section of a human kidney. Half the kidney has been sliced away. Note that the structure shows regional differences. The outer portion (cortex) contains all the glomeruli. The collecting ducts form a large portion of the inner kidney (medulla), giving it a striped, pyramid-like appearance, and these drain into the renal pelvis. The papilla is the inner portion of the medulla.

and an **inner zone,** including the papilla. All these distinctions reflect the arrangement of the various components of the microscopic subunits of the kidneys, to which we now turn.

The Nephron

In humans, each kidney is made up of approximately one million tiny units called **nephrons,** one of which is shown diagrammatically in Fig. 1-3. Each nephron consists of a filtering component, called the **renal corpuscle,** and a **tubule** extending from the renal corpuscle.[4] Let us begin with the renal corpus-

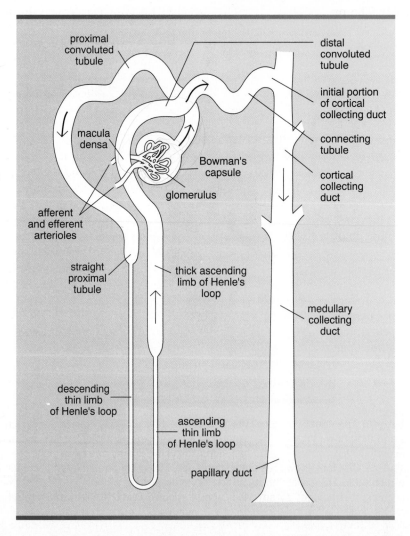

Fig. 1-3   Relationships of component parts of a long-looped nephron, which has been "uncoiled" for clarity (relative lengths of the different segments are not drawn to scale). The combination of glomerulus and Bowman's capsule is the renal corpuscle.

cle, which is responsible for the initial step in urine formation, the separation of a protein-free filtrate from plasma.

The Renal Corpuscle

  The renal corpuscle consists of a compact tuft of interconnected capillary loops, the **glomerulus** (plural = glomeruli) or **glomerular capillaries,** and a balloonlike hollow capsule, **Bowman's capsule,** into which the glomerulus protrudes (Fig. 1-4). One way of visualizing the relationship between the glomerulus and Bowman's capsule is to imagine a loosely clenched fist (the glomerulus) punched into a balloon (Bowman's capsule). The part of Bowman's capsule in contact with the glomerulus becomes pushed inward but does not make contact with the opposite side of the capsule; accordingly, a space (the **urinary space** or **Bowman's space**) exists within the capsule, and it is into this space that fluid filters.

  This filtration barrier in the renal corpuscle consists of three layers: the capillary endothelium of the glomerular capillaries, a basement membrane, and the single-celled layer of epithelial cells constituting Bowman's capsule (Fig. 1-4). The first layer, the endothelial cells of the capillaries, is perforated by many large fenestrae ("windows"). The basement membrane is a gel-like acellular meshwork of glycoproteins and proteoglycans.[5] The capsular epithelial cells that rest on the basement membrane are called **podocytes**. They are quite different from the relatively simple, flattened cells that line the rest of Bowman's capsule (the part of the "balloon" not in contact with the "fist"). The podocytes have an unusual octopuslike structure in that they possess a large number of extensions, or **foot processes,** which are embedded in the basement membrane. The foot processes from adjacent podocytes manifest a great degree of interdigitation. **Slits** between adjacent foot processes constitute the path through which the filtrate, once through the endothelial cells and basement membrane, travels to enter Bowman's space. However, for two reasons, these slits do not offer completely open passageways: (1) The foot processes are coated by a thick layer of extracellular material (glycosialoproteins), which partially occludes the slits; (2) extremely thin diaphragms bridge the slits at the surface of the basement membrane.

  The functional significance of this anatomical arrangement is that blood in the glomerulus is separated from Bowman's space by only a thin set of membranes, which permit the filtration of fluid from the capillaries into the space. Bowman's capsule connects at the side opposite the glomerulus with the first portion of the tubule, into which this filtered fluid then flows.

  Our discussion of the renal corpuscle has focused on the two types of cells—capillary endothelium and podocytes—in the filtration barrier. There is a third cell type—**mesangial cells**—found in the central part of the glomerulus between and within capillary loops. Some of the glomerular mesangial cells act as phagocytes, whereas most contain large numbers of myofilaments and can contract in response to a variety of stimuli. The role such contraction plays in influencing filtration by the renal corpuscles will be discussed in Chapter 2.

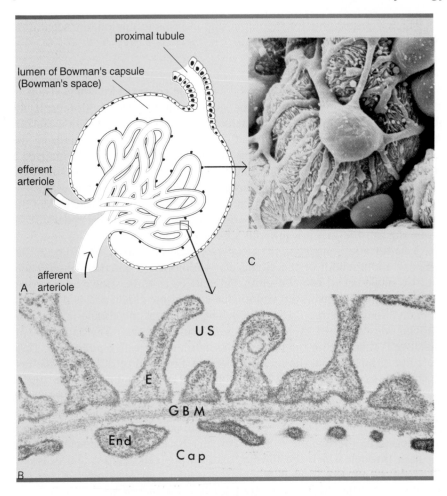

Fig. 1-4 (*A*) Anatomy of the glomerulus. (*B*) Cross section of glomerular membranes. US = "urinary" (Bowman's) space; E = epithelial foot processes; GBM = glomerular basement membranes; End = capillary endothelium; Cap = lumen of capillary. Note the slit diaphragms covering the basement membrane between foot processes. (*Courtesy HG Rennke; originally published in* Fed Proc *1977;36:2019; reprinted with permission.*) (*C*) Scanning electron micrograph of podocytes covering glomerular capillary loops; the view is from inside Bowman's space. The large mass is a cell body. Note the remarkable interdigitation of the foot processes from adjacent podocytes and the slits between them. (*Courtesy Dr. Craig Tisher.*)

The Tubule   Throughout its course, the tubule is made up of a single layer of epithelial cells resting on a basement membrane. The structural and immunocytochemical characteristics of these epithelial cells vary from segment to segment of the tubule, but one common feature is the presence of tight junctions between adjacent cells.

The left portion of Table 1-2 lists the names and sequence of the various tubular segments, as illustrated in Figs. 1-3 and 1-5. Physiologists and anatomists have traditionally grouped two or more contiguous tubular segments for purposes of reference, but the terminologies have varied considerably. The right half of Table 1-2 gives the combination terms this book will use.[6]

The proximal tubule, which drains Bowman's capsule, consists of a coiled segment—the **proximal convoluted tubule**—followed by a straight segment—the **proximal straight tubule**—which descends toward the medulla.

The next segment, into which the proximal straight tubule drains, is the **descending thin limb of Henle's loop** (or simply the descending thin limb). The descending thin limb ends at a hairpin loop, and the tubule then begins to ascend parallel to the descending limb. In long loops (see below), the epithelium of the first portion of this ascending limb remains thin, although different from that of the descending limb, and this segment is called the **ascending thin limb of Henle's loop** (or simply the ascending thin limb) (Fig. 1-5). Beyond this segment, in these long loops, the epithelium thickens and this next segment is called the **thick ascending limb of Henle's loop** (or simply the thick ascending limb). In short loops (see below), there is no ascending thin limb and the thick ascending limb begins right at the hairpin loop (Fig. 1-5).

Near the end of every thick ascending limb, the tubule passes between the arterioles supplying its renal corpuscle of origin (see Fig. 1-3). This very short segment—really a plaque in the wall of the thick ascending limb—is known as the **macula densa**. A little beyond the macula densa, the thick ascending limb ends and the **distal convoluted tubule** begins. This is followed by the **connecting tubule**, which leads to the **cortical collecting duct**, the first portion of which is called the *initial collecting tubule*.

In the great majority of cases, from Bowman's capsule to the initial collecting tubules, each of the one million nephrons in each kidney is completely separate from the others. A number of initial collecting tubules then join end to end or side to side to form larger cortical collecting ducts. All the cortical

Table 1-2 Terminology for the Tubular Segments

Sequence of segments	Combination terms used in text
Proximal convoluted tubule Proximal straight tubule	Proximal tubule
Descending thin limb of Henle's loop Ascending thin limb of Henle's loop Thick ascending limb of Henle's loop (contains macula densa near end)	Henle's loop
Distal convoluted tubule	
Connecting tubule Cortical collecting duct Outer medullary collecting duct Inner medullary collecting duct (last portion is papillary duct)	Collecting-duct system

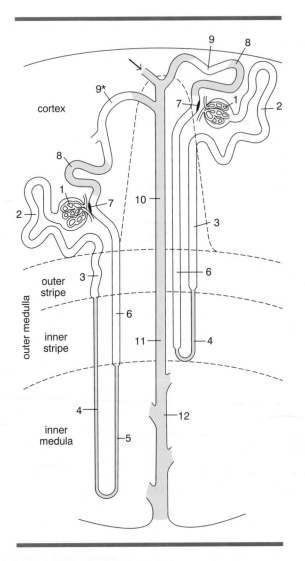

Fig. 1-5 Standard nomenclature for structures of the kidney (1988 Commission of the International Union of Physiological Sciences). Shown are a short-looped and a long-looped (juxtamedullary) nephron, together with the collecting system (not drawn to scale). A cortical medullary ray—the part of the cortex that contains the straight proximal tubules, cortical thick ascending limbs, and cortical collecting ducts—is delineated by a dashed line. 1, renal corpuscle (Bowman's capsule and the glomerulus); 2, proximal convoluted tubule; 3, proximal straight tubule; 4, descending thin limb; 5, ascending thin limb; 6, thick ascending limb; 7, macula densa (located within the final portion of the thick ascending limb); 8, distal convoluted tubule; 9, connecting tubule; 9*, connecting tubule of a juxtamedullary nephron that arches upward to form a so-called arcade (there are only a few of these in the human kidney); 10, cortical collecting duct; 11, outer medullary collecting duct; 12, inner medullary collecting duct. See Table 1-2 for additional terms used in the text to denote combinations of two or more contiguous tubular segments. (*From W Kriz and L Bankir,* Am J Physiol *1988; 254LF:F1-F8; with permission.*)

collecting ducts then run downward to enter the medulla and become **outer medullary collecting ducts** and then **inner medullary collecting ducts**. The latter merge to form several hundred large ducts, the last portions of which are called *papillary collecting ducts,* each of which empties into a calyx of the renal pelvis.

Each renal pelvis is continuous with a **ureter**, which empties into the **urinary bladder**, where urine is temporarily stored and from which it is intermittently eliminated. The urine is not altered after it enters a calyx. From this point on, the remainder of the urinary system serves simply as plumbing.

As noted earlier, the tubular epithelium is one cell thick throughout. Before the distal convoluted tubule, the cells in any given segment are homogeneous and distinct for that segment. Thus, for example, the thick ascending limb contains only *thick ascending limb cells*. However, beginning in the second half of the distal convoluted tubule *two* cell types are found in most of the remaining segments. One type constitutes the majority of cells in the particular segment, is considered specific for that segment, and is named accordingly— *distal convoluted tubule cells*, *connecting tubule cells*, and *collecting duct cells*, the last known more commonly as **principal cells**. Interspersed among the segment-specific cells in each of these three segments are individual cells of the second type, called **intercalated cells**. To make things still more complicated, we shall see that there are actually two types of intercalated cells—type A and type B.[7] (The last portion of the medullary collecting duct contains neither principal cells nor intercalated cells but is composed entirely of a distinct cell type called the *inner medullary collecting duct cells.*)

Several simplifying conventions will be used in this book: (1) I will not usually distinguish between the convoluted and straight portions of the proximal tubule; (2) the functioning of the connecting tubule is generally similar to that of the cortical collecting duct, and I will always tacitly include the former segment when I describe the latter; and (3) neither the cortical collecting duct nor the medullary collecting duct is a structurally or functionally homogeneous structure (e.g., note the last sentence in the previous paragraph), but except where particularly relevant I will treat each as though it were.

Blood Supply to the Nephrons

In the earlier section on the renal corpuscle, I described the glomerulus but made no mention of the origin of these capillaries. Blood enters each kidney via a renal artery, which then divides into progressively smaller branches— interlobar, arcuate, and finally cortical radial arteries (formerly called interlobular arteries). Each of the cortical radial arteries gives off at right angles to itself, as it courses toward the outer kidney surface, a parallel series of **afferent arterioles** (Figs. 1-3 and 1-6), each of which leads to a glomerulus. (Thus, the afferent arteriole is the "arm" to which the "fist" is attached.)

Normally only about 20 percent of the plasma (and none of the erythrocytes) entering the glomerulus is filtered from the glomerulus into Bowman's capsule. Where does the remaining blood go next? In almost all other organs, capillaries recombine to form the beginnings of the venous system, but the

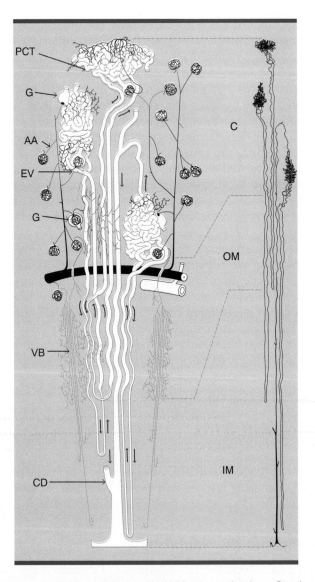

Fig. 1-6 Diagram of renal vascular and tubular organization. On the left, three nephrons (one from each general population) are shown; their vascular structures are extensively simplified, and vertical scale is compressed. The same nephrons are shown undistorted to the right. Major zones are cortex (C), outer medulla (OM), and inner medulla (IM). Afferent arterioles (AA), glomeruli (G), and efferent vessels (EV) are shown together with part of the peritubular capillary network. The proximal convoluted tubules (PCT) and distal convoluted tubules (dark hatching) are generally dissociated from the efferent network arising from their parent glomeruli. Some midcortical efferents directly perfuse loops of Henle and collecting ducts in cortical medullary rays. In outer medulla, descending thin limbs of short loops are close to vascular bundles (VB), and thin limbs of long loops are found with thick ascending limbs and collecting ducts (CD) in the interbundle region. (*Courtesy Reiner Beeuwks III; adapted from* Am J Physiol *1975; 229:695.*)

glomerular capillaries instead recombine to form another set of arterioles called the **efferent arterioles**. Thus, blood leaves each glomerulus through a single efferent arteriole (Fig. 1-4), which soon subdivides into a second set of capillaries (Fig. 1-6). These are the **peritubular capillaries**, which are profusely distributed to the tubule. The peritubular capillaries then rejoin to form the veins by which blood ultimately leaves the kidney.

The vascular structures supplying the medulla also differ from those in the cortex (Fig. 1-6). From many of the juxtamedullary glomeruli, long efferent arterioles extend to the outer medulla, where they divide many times to form **vascular bundles.** The margins of these bundles give rise to a capillary network that surrounds Henle's loops and the collecting ducts in the outer medulla. From the cores of the bundles, straight vessels (**descending vasa recta**) extend to the inner medulla, where they also break up into a capillary plexus. These inner medullary capillaries re-form into veins (**ascending vasa recta**) that run in close association with the descending vasa recta within the vascular bundles. This relationship, as we shall see, has significance for the formation of concentrated urine.

Categories of Nephrons

There are important regional differences in the various tubular segments of the nephron. The cortex contains all the renal corpuscles (this accounts for its granular appearance), convoluted portions of the proximal tubule, cortical portions of Henle's loops, distal convoluted tubules, connecting tubules, and cortical collecting ducts. The medulla contains the medullary portions of Henle's loops and the medullary collecting ducts.

Nephrons are categorized according to the locations of their renal corpuscles in the cortex (Fig. 1-5): (1) In **superficial cortical nephrons** renal corpuscles are located within 1 mm of the capsular surface of the kidneys; (2) in **midcortical nephrons** renal corpuscles are located, as their name implies, in the midcortex, deep to the superficial cortical nephrons but above the next category; (3) in **juxtamedullary nephrons** renal corpuscles are located just above the junction between cortex and medulla. One major distinction among these three categories is the length of Henle's loop. All superficial cortical nephrons have short loops, which make their hairpin turn above the junction of outer and inner medulla. All juxtamedullary nephrons have long loops, which extend into the inner medulla, often to the tip of a papilla. Midcortical nephrons may be either short-looped or long-looped. The additional length of Henle's loop in long-looped nephrons is due to a longer descending thin limb and the presence of an ascending thin limb. Finally, the beginning of the thick ascending limb in the longest loops marks the border between outer and inner medulla; in other words, the thick ascending limbs are found only in the cortex and outer medulla.

Nephron Heterogeneity

As stated earlier, there are more than two million nephrons in the two human kidneys. These nephrons manifest significant differences in anatomical, biochemical, and functional characteristics beyond those described in the previous section. For simplicity, however, I will generally ignore these complexities, many of which are not fully understood at present.[8]

The Juxtaglomerular Apparatus

Reference was made earlier to the macula densa, a portion of the late thick ascending limb at the point where, in all nephrons, this segment courses between the afferent and efferent arterioles at the hilum of the renal corpuscle of its own nephron. This entire area is known as the **juxtaglomerular (JG) apparatus** (Fig. 1-7). (Don't confuse the term *juxtaglomerular apparatus* with *juxtamedullary nephron*.) Each JG apparatus is made up of three cell types: (1) **granular cells,** which are differentiated smooth muscle cells in the walls of the arterioles, particularly in the afferent arterioles; (2) extraglomerular mesangial cells; and (3) macula densa cells.

The granular cells (so called because they contain secretory vesicles) are the cells that secrete the hormone renin, mentioned earlier in this chapter. The extraglomerular mesangial cells are morphologically similar to and continuous with the glomerular mesangial cells. The macula densa contributes to the control of glomerular filtration rate and to the control of renin secretion (Chapter 2).

Renal Innervation

The kidneys receive a rich supply of sympathetic noradrenergic neurons. These are distributed to the afferent and efferent arterioles, the juxtaglomerular apparatus, and many portions of the tubule. There is no significant parasympathetic innnervation. There are some dopamine-containing neurons, the functions of which are uncertain.

INTRODUCTION TO BASIC RENAL PROCESSES

The three basic renal processes are known as glomerular filtration, tubular reabsorption, and tubular secretion. This section will merely introduce these processes, which will be discussed in detail in Chapters 2 and 4. Keep in mind as you go through this section that the kidneys work only on plasma; the erythrocytes supply oxygen to the kidneys but serve no other function in urine formation.

Glomerular Filtration

Urine formation begins with **glomerular filtration**, the bulk-flow of fluid from the glomerular capillaries into Bowman's capsule. The **glomerular filtrate**, i.e., the fluid within Bowman's capsule, normally contains no cells, is essentially protein-free, and contains most inorganic ions and low-molecular-weight organic solutes (glucose and amino acids, for example) in virtually the same concentrations as in the plasma.

The volume of filtrate formed per unit time is known as the **glomerular filtration rate, GFR**. In a normal young adult male, the GFR is an incredible

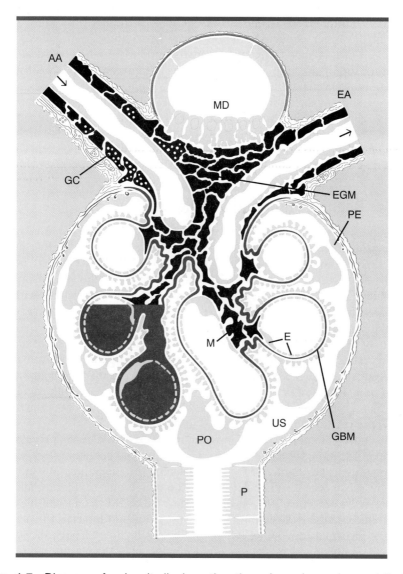

Fig. 1-7 Diagram of a longitudinal section through a glomerulus and its juxtaglomerular apparatus. The juxtaglomerular apparatus consists of the granular cells (GC), which secrete renin, the macula densa (MD), and the extraglomerular mesangial cells (EGM). E = endothelium of the capillaries; EA = efferent arteriole; AA = afferent arteriole; PE = parietal (outer) epithelium of Bowman's capsule; P = proximal tubular cells; US = urinary (Bowman's) space; PO = podocytes of Bowman's capsule; GBM = glomerular basement membrane. (*From W Kriz et al. in: Davidson, AM, ed.* Proceedings of the 10th International Congress on Nephrology, Vol. 1; *London: Balliere Tindall; 1987:3-23.*)

180 L/day (125 ml/min)![9] (Contrast this value with the net filtration of fluid across all the other capillaries in the body—approximately 4 L/day.) The implications of this huge GFR are extremely important. When we recall that the average total volume of plasma in humans is approximately 3 L, it follows that the entire plasma volume is filtered by the kidneys some 60 times a day. The opportunity to filter such huge volumes of plasma enables the kidneys to excrete large quantities of waste products and to regulate the constituents of the internal environment very precisely.

The forces that determine the GFR and their physiological control will be described in Chapters 2 and 7.

Tubular Reabsorption and Tubular Secretion

The volume and solute content of the final urine which enters the renal pelvis is quite different from those of the glomerular filtrate. That is because as the filtrate flows from Bowman's capsule through the various portions of the tubule its composition is altered by two general processes: tubular reabsorption and tubular secretion. The tubule is at all points intimately associated with the peritubular capillaries, a relationship that permits transfer of materials between the peritubular-capillary plasma and the lumen of the tubule. When the direction of transfer is from tubular lumen to peritubular-capillary plasma, the process is called **tubular reabsorption** (also called *absorption*[10]). Movement in the opposite direction, i.e., from peritubular-capillary plasma to tubular lumen, is called **tubular secretion.** This last term must not be confused with **excretion**. To say that a substance has been excreted is to say that it appears in the final urine. These relationships are illustrated in Fig. 1-8.

The most common relationships among these basic renal processes—glomerular filtration, tubular reabsorption, and tubular secretion—are shown in the hypothetical examples of Fig. 1-9. Plasma, containing three low-molecular-weight substances X, Y, and Z, enters the glomerular capillaries, and approximately 20 percent of the plasma is filtered into Bowman's capsule. The filtrate, which contains X, Y, and Z in the same concentrations as the plasma, enters the proximal convoluted tubule and begins its flow through the rest of the tubule. Simultaneously, the remaining 80 percent of the plasma, with its X, Y, and Z, leaves the glomerular capillaries via the efferent arterioles and enters the peritubular capillaries. The cells of the tubular epithelium can secrete all the peritubular-capillary X into the tubular lumen but cannot reabsorb X. Thus, by the combination of filtration and tubular secretion, all the plasma that originally entered the renal artery is cleared of substance X, which leaves the body via the urine. The tubule can reabsorb Y and Z. The amount of Y reabsorption is small, so most of the filtered Y is not reabsorbed and escapes from the body in the urine. But for Z the reabsorptive mechanism is so powerful that virtually all the filtered Z is reabsorbed. Therefore, no Z is lost from the body. Hence, the processes of filtration and reabsorption have canceled each other, and the net result is as though Z had never entered the kidney at all.

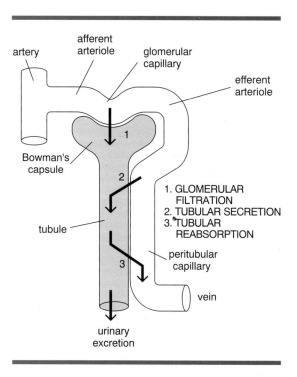

Fig. 1-8 The three basic renal processes. This figure illustrates only the directions of reabsorption and secretion, not specific sites or order of occurrence. Depending on the specific substance, reabsorption and secretion can occur at various sites along the tubule.

As we shall see, many more substances undergo tubular reabsorption than tubular secretion. An idea of the magnitude and importance of tubular reabsorption can be gained from Table 1-3, which summarizes data for a few plasma components that undergo reabsorption. The values in Table 1-3 are typical for a normal person on an average diet. There are at least three important generalizations to be drawn from this table:

1. Because of the huge GFR the filtered quantities are enormous, generally larger than the amounts of the substances in the body. For example, the body contains about 40 L of water, but the volume of water filtered each day is 180 L. If reabsorption of water ceased but filtration continued, the total plasma water would be urinated within 30 min.
2. Reabsorption of waste products, such as urea, is relatively incomplete, so that large fractions of their filtered amounts are excreted in the urine, like substance Y in our hypothetical example.
3. Reabsorption of most "useful" plasma components, e.g., water, electrolytes, and glucose, is relatively complete, so that the amounts excreted in the urine represent very small fractions of the filtered amounts.

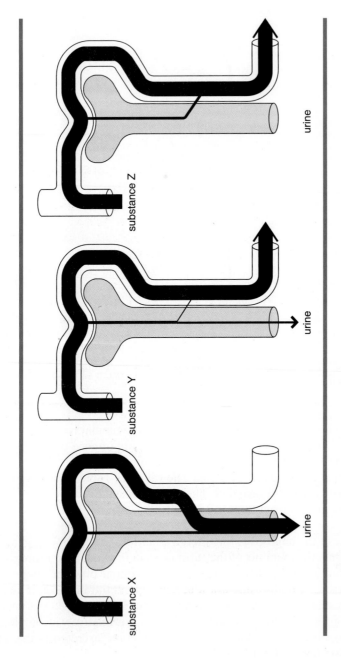

Fig. 1-9   Renal manipulation of three hypothetical substances, X, Y, and Z. X is filtered and secreted but not reabsorbed. Y is filtered, and a fraction is then reabsorbed. Z is filtered but is completely reabsorbed.

Table 1-3 Average Values for Several Substances Handled by Filtration and Reabsorption

Substance	Amount filtered per day	Amount excreted	% reabsorbed
Water, L	180	1.8	99.0
Sodium, g	630	3.2	99.5
Glucose, g	180	0	100
Urea, g	56	28	50

For each plasma substance a particular combination of filtration, reabsorption, and secretion applies, i.e., all three processes do not necessarily apply to every substance. A critical point is that the rates at which the relevant processes proceed for many of these substances are subject to physiological control. By triggering changes in the rates of filtration, reabsorption, or secretion when the body content of a substance goes above or below normal, homeostatic mechanisms can regulate the substance's bodily balance. For example, consider what happens when a person drinks a lot of water: Within 1 to 2 h all the excess water has been excreted in the urine, partly as the result of an increase in GFR but mainly as the result of decreased tubular reabsorption of water. In this example, the kidney is the effector organ of a reflex that maintains body water concentration within very narrow limits.

In summary, one can study the normal renal handling of any given substance by asking a series of questions:

1. To what degree is the substance filterable at the renal corpuscle?
2. Is it reabsorbed?
3. Is it secreted?
4. What are the mechanisms by which reabsorption or secretion is achieved?
5. What factors homeostatically regulate the quantities filtered, reabsorbed, or secreted: i.e., what are the pathways by which renal excretion of the substance is altered to maintain stable body balance?
6. What factors other than renal disease can perturb body balance by causing the kidneys to filter, reabsorb, or secrete too much or too little of the substance?

Clinicians, of course, must ask a seventh question: How do the various types of renal disease influence the handling of the substance and its total-body balance?

Metabolism by the Tubules

Although renal physiologists traditionally list glomerular filtration, tubular reabsorption, and tubular secretion as the three basic renal processes, a fourth process—metabolism by the tubular cells—is also of considerable importance

for some substances. For example, the tubular cells may extract organic nutrients from the glomerular filtrate or peritubular capillaries and metabolize
them as dictated by the cells' own nutrient requirements. In so doing, the renal
cells are behaving no differently than any other cells in the body. In contrast,
other metabolic transformations performed by the kidney are not directed
toward its own nutritional requirements but rather toward altering the composition of the urine and plasma. The most important of these are the synthesis
of ammonium from glutamine and the production of bicarbonate, both described in Chapter 9.

INTRARENAL CHEMICAL MESSENGERS

In response to appropriate stimuli, the kidneys themselves synthesize a large
number of substances that function within the kidneys as local chemical messengers, that is, as paracrine or autocrine agents (another name for both groups
is *autacoids*). Those with the best documented functions, described in Chapters
2 and 7, are angiotensin II and the eicosanoids.

As described earlier in this chapter, **angiotensin II** functions as a *hormone*
in that it reaches its target organs, including the kidneys, via the arterial blood.
However, because the kidneys produce renin and because renal tissue also
contains both angiotensinogen and angiotensin-converting enzyme, the reactions generating angiotensin II can occur completely within the kidneys. Accordingly, the kidneys are influenced not only by blood-borne angiotensin II
but also by angiotensin II produced intrarenally and acting, therefore, as a
paracrine agent.

Eicosanoid is a general term that includes all the oxygenated derivatives
of arachidonic acid metabolism. The vascular endothelium and epithelial cells
of several tubular segments produce many prostaglandins, including PGE_2 and
PGI_2 (prostacyclin), as well as thromboxane A_2 (TXA_2) and leukotrienes.

Other intrarenal paracrine agents are listed, *for reference,* in Table 1-4;
postulated functions for some of them will be given in subsequent chapters.
The interested reader may obtain more information by consulting the Suggested Readings. This is also a good time to remind you about the use of the
objectives at the beginning of each chapter. You will note that the last objective
of this chapter deals with angiotensin II and the eicosanoids, but not with the
other messengers of Table 1-4; the objectives always tell you exactly what
factual material I think you should learn.

METHODS IN RENAL PHYSIOLOGY

Because of its limited scope and objectives, this book will deal very little with
the methods used to study renal physiology. Only the method known as *clearance* is described to any extent (in Chapter 3) because of its widespread clinical
use. Another technique that has been a mainstay of renal physiologists is
micropuncture, the insertion of a micropipette into a nephron segment to

Table 1-4   Some Intrarenal Paracrine Agents

Angiotensin II See text

Eicosanoids See text

Kinins
This is the collective name given to the peptides released from specific plasma protein precursors—*kininogens*—by several plasma and tissue enzymes called *kallikreins*. The specific kallikrein produced and secreted by the kidneys (by cells of distal tubular segments) splits plasma kininogen to yield *lysl bradykinin,* which is cleaved again within the kidneys to yield *bradykinin* (note the biochemical analogies between the kallikrein-kinin and renin-angiotensin systems). Bradykinin can exert potent effects on the renal vasculature (Chapter 2), renin secretion, and ion transport, but its precise physiological function in the kidneys remains unclear.

Dopamine
It was mentioned in the text that some of the renal nerves may release dopamine. In addition, the tubules produce dopamine, which may influence the renal vasculature (Chapter 2), as well as ion transport (Chapter 7).

Endothelin
This term denotes a family of homologous 21-amino-acid peptides having very widespread distribution in the body. In the kidneys endothelin is secreted by the vascular endothelium and cells of several tubular segments, and is a potent vasoconstrictor (Chapter 2).

Growth Factors
The kidneys produce and respond locally to a large number of growth factors (for example, insulin-like growth factor 1). These messengers cause the increase in renal size and changes in development that occur in a variety of situations, including embryogenesis and compensatory renal hypertrophy—the increase in kidney growth that follows loss of part or all of a kidney. They may also influence other aspects of renal function.

Adenosine
This metabolite, produced by the renal tubules and probably other renal cells helps regulate the rates of filtration in the renal corpuscles and renin secretion (Chapter 2).

Endothelium-derived relaxing factor (EDRF)
The vascular endothelium of the kidneys, like that of many other tissues and organs, produces EDRF, now identified as *nitric oxide*, which is known to be a vasodilator in many vascular beds, including the kidneys (Chapter 2).

Cytokines
Lymphocytes and macrophages within the kidneys secrete the same huge battery of cytokines (e.g., interleukin 1) secreted elsewhere by these cells. These cytokines not only mediate immune function intrarenally but may also influence the renal vasculature and tubules under normal physiological conditions.

withdraw fluid for analysis and to measure pressures, perfuse tubules, and perform other manipulations on single nephrons in situ. A third technique is that of perfusing isolated separated segments of a single nephron in vitro.

In addition to clearance, micropuncture, and the isolated, perfused tubule, a plethora of other useful techniques, including those of molecular biology, have been developed. The interested reader should consult the Suggested Readings.

Study questions: 1 to 4

NOTES

[1]However, the kidneys are not the major regulators of *all* essential inorganic substances. In particular, the bodily balances of many of the trace elements, such as zinc and iron, are regulated mainly by control of gastrointestinal absorption of the element or by control of biliary secretion. This statement, in large part, is also true of calcium. Nevertheless, even for these elements some renal excretion occurs and may constitute an important source of bodily imbalance in various diseases.

[2]It is likely that the oxygen sensor in the interstitial cells is a rapidly turning over heme protein whose configuration changes when oxygen binds to it.

[3]The biochemistry of the renin-angiotensin system is actually far more complex than the description shown in Fig. 1-1 and described in the text. Just a few of the important additional findings are as follows: (1) Approximately half the renin in plasma is the inactive prohormone form of renin (prorenin) initially synthesized by the kidneys, and it is possible that this protein can be activated to renin by enzymes in peripheral tissues; (2) clinically important situations exist in which changes in the concentrations of angiotensinogen or angiotensin-converting enzyme occur, which may significantly increase or reduce the generation of angiotensin II at any given plasma concentration of renin (e.g., oral contraceptives may cause a large increase in plasma angiotensinogen, whereas lung disease may reduce angiotensin-converting enzyme activity in the pulmonary capillaries); and (3) in several tissues an enzyme exists which splits angiotensin II to yield the heptapeptide known as angiotensin III, which is also active biologically, although its relative contribution compared with that of angiotensin II is probably small.

[4]Strictly speaking, the last portions of the tubule, the collecting-duct system, are not part of the nephron, but for simplicity renal physiologists generally ignore this fact, a policy we shall follow.

[5]The glomerular basement membrane is formed by the merging, during development, of distinct capillary and epithelial-cell basement membranes. This fact has relevance for certain kidney diseases.

[6]For anyone who wishes to read further in the literature of renal physiology, a few more words about terminology may be helpful. A recent attempt to standardize combination terms for contiguous tubular segments (see Kriz and Bankir in Suggested Readings) recommended the use of *proximal tubule* and *collecting-duct system* adopted in this book. However, it also recommended *intermediate tubule* to refer to both the descending and ascending thin limbs of Henle's loop, and *distal tubule* for the combination of the thick ascending limb of Henle's loop and the distal convoluted tubule. These two recommendations have not been adopted by most renal physiologists and are not used in this book. Moreover, the term *distal tubule* is particularly confusing in the literature,

both past and present: Anatomists have used it as defined in the recommendation above, but for physiologists it has denoted that portion of the tubule extending from the region of the macula densa to the first junction with another tubule. This includes, therefore, the distal convoluted tubule, the connecting tubule, and the initial collecting tubule; in this usage, the distal convoluted tubule was called the *early distal tubule* and the other two segments the *late distal tubule.* To avoid confusion, I have chosen not to use *distal tubule* at all in this book.

[7]Another characteristic of the segments beyond the thick ascending limb is transitional zones in which the segment-specific cell types of adjacent segments are somewhat intermingled so that precise delineation of the beginning and end of segments becomes a matter of definition.

[8]Actually the term *nephron heterogeneity* has come to have two distinct meanings, the first being the one given in the text and the second denoting the differences between the various tubular segments in a single nephron. (See Hebert, and Sands et al. in Suggested Readings, Analysis of Individual Nephron Segments.)

[9]This value is slightly lower in women and declines with age in both sexes, because of a decrease in the number of functioning nephrons.

[10]*Absorption* has come into more recent usage and is really the more accurate term since *reabsorption* literally means "absorption again," a misleading concept. However, we have chosen to continue to use *reabsorption* since it is the original time-honored term and is still the more commonly used of the two.

RENAL BLOOD FLOW AND GLOMERULAR FILTRATION

Objectives

The student understands the relationships between flow, resistance, and pressure in the kidneys:

1 Defines RBF, RPF, GFR, and filtration fraction, and gives normal values
2 States the formula relating flow, pressure, and resistance in an organ
3 Describes, in qualitative terms, the relative resistances of the afferent arterioles and efferent arterioles
4 Describes the effects of changes in afferent- and efferent-arteriolar resistances on renal blood flow

The student understands how glomerular filtrate is formed and the forces that determine its rate of formation:

1 Describes how molecular size and electrical charge determine filterability of plasma solutes; states how protein-binding of a low-molecular-weight substance influences its filterability
2 States the formula for the determinants of glomerular filtration rate, and states, in qualitative terms, why the net filtration pressure is positive; defines hydraulic permeability and filtration coefficient (K_f)
3 States how mesangial cells might alter K_f; states the reason GFR is so large relative to filtration across other capillaries in the body
4 Describes how arterial pressure, afferent-arteriolar resistance, and efferent-arteriolar resistance determine glomerular-capillary pressure
5 States the effect of obstruction on P_{BC}
6 Describes how changes in renal plasma flow influence average Π_{GC}

The student understands the normal controls of RBF and GFR:

1 Defines autoregulation of RBF and GFR; states the condition in which "pure" autoregulation can be observed; states the adaptive function of autoregulation
2 Describes the myogenic and tubuloglomerular feedback mechanisms of autoregulation
3 States how tubuloglomerular feedback lowers GFR when proximal reabsorption is inhibited
4 Describes the direct effects of the renal sympathetic nerves on renal arterioles and how these effects influence RBF and GFR
5 States the reflexes that cause renal sympathetic nerve activity to increase; describes the adaptive value of this increase
6 States the effects of angiotensin II on renal arterioles and glomerular K_f and how these effects influence RBF and GFR
7 Describes the four major controls of renin secretion; identifies the type of adrenergic receptor involved in the direct sympathetic pathway
8 States the adaptive value of the increased renin secretion triggered by low arterial blood pressure
9 States the effect of the renal nerves and angiotension II on renal prostaglandin synthesis and the function served by the prostaglandins
10 Given the effects of a messenger or drug on the afferent and efferent arterioles, predicts the effects of the agent on RBF and GFR

The **renal blood flow (RBF)** in a typical adult is approximately 1.1 L/min. Thus, the kidneys receive 20 to 25 percent of the total cardiac output (5 L/min) even though their combined weight is less than 1 percent of total-body weight. Given a normal hematocrit of 0.45, the **renal plasma flow (RPF)** = 0.55 × 1.1 L/min = 605 ml/min. As stated in Chapter 1 the **glomerular filtration rate (GFR)** is 125 ml/min. Thus, of the 605 ml of plasma that enters the glomeruli via the afferent arterioles, 125/605, or 20 percent, filters into Bowman's capsule, the remaining 480 ml passing via the efferent arterioles into the peritubular capillaries. This ratio—GFR/RPF—is known as the **filtration fraction.**

FLOW, RESISTANCE, AND PRESSURE IN THE KIDNEYS

The basic equation for blood flow through any organ is:

$$\text{Organ blood flow} = \Delta P/R \qquad (2\text{-}1)$$

where ΔP = mean arterial pressure minus venous pressure for that organ, and R = total vascular resistance in that organ. Resistance is determined by the blood viscosity and the lengths and radii of the organ's blood vessels, the arteriolar radii being overwhelmingly the major contributors. These radii are determined by the state of contraction of the arteriolar smooth muscle.

The existence of two sets of arterioles and two sets of capillaries—the glomeruli and the peritubular capillaries—makes the renal vasculature unusual. Normally, the resistances of the afferent arterioles and efferent arterioles are approximately equal and account for most of the total renal vascular resistance. Because the two capillary beds are separated by the efferent arterioles, the hydraulic (also called hydrostatic) pressure in the second bed—the peritubular capillaries—is much lower than in the first—the glomeruli (20 mmHg vs 60 mmHg, in a normal unstressed individual). As we shall see, the high glomerular pressure is crucial for glomerular filtration (this chapter), whereas the low peritubular-capillary pressure is equally crucial for the tubular reabsorption of fluid (Chapter 6).

To repeat, the RBF is determined mainly by the mean arterial pressure and the contractile state of the smooth muscle of the renal arterioles. Now for a simple but very important point: *A given change in arteriolar resistance produces the same effect on RBF regardless of whether it occurs in the afferent arteriole or efferent arteriole.* When the two resistances both change in the same direction, the most common state of affairs, their effects on RBF will be additive (since the two resistances are in series). When they change in different directions—one resistance increasing and the other decreasing—they exert opposing effects on RBF. We shall see in the next section that *the story is totally different for GFR.*

It should also be emphasized that the renal cortex receives the great majority of the renal blood flow (normally more than 90 percent). The paucity of medullary blood flow (its adaptive value for urine concentration will be discussed in Chapter 7) is due to the high resistance offered by the vasa recta. Blood flows in the cortex and medulla are subject to a degree of independent control, and this chapter will deal only with the cortical vasculature (see Chou et al. and Pallone et al. in Suggested Readings for a description of the medullary circulation and its control).

GLOMERULAR FILTRATION

Formation of Glomerular Filtrate

As stated in Chapter 1 the glomerular filtrate is essentially protein-free and contains most inorganic ions and low-molecular-weight organic solutes in virtually the same concentrations as in the plasma.[1] (The reasons for the qualifying terms "essentially" and "most" in this last sentence will be described shortly.)

The route that filtered substances take through the membranes of a renal corpuscle is as follows: fenestrae in the glomerular-capillary endothelial layer, basement membrane, slit diaphragms, and slits between podocyte foot processes. Just which of these structures constitute the major barriers to filtration of macromolecules has proven a difficult question to answer,[2] but it is clear that they do so on the basis of both molecular size and electrical charge. Let us look first at size.

The membranes of the renal corpuscle provide no hindrance at all to the movement of molecules with molecular weights less than 7000 and almost total hindrance to plasma albumin (molecular weight approximately 70,000). (We are, for simplicity, using molecular weight as our reference for size; in reality it is molecular radius that is critical.) The hindrance to plasma albumin is not 100 percent, however, and so the glomerular filtrate does contain extremely small quantities of albumin, on the order of 10 mg/L or less. This is only about 0.02 percent of the concentration of albumin in plasma and is the reason for the use of the phrase "essentially protein-free" in the first paragraph of this section.

For molecules between 7000 and 70,000, filterability becomes progressively smaller as the molecule becomes larger. Thus, many normally occurring plasma peptides and small proteins are filtered to a significant degree. Moreover, when certain small proteins not normally present in the plasma appear because of disease (e.g., hemoglobin released from damaged erythrocytes, and myoglobin released from damaged muscles), considerable filtration of these may occur.

Electrical charge is the second variable determining filterability of macromolecules. For any given size, negatively charged macromolecules are filtered to a lesser extent, and positively charged macromolecules to a greater extent, than neutral molecules. The reason is that the surfaces of all the components of the filtration barrier (the cell coats of the endothelium, the basement membrane, and the cell coats of the podocytes) contain fixed polyanions, which repel negatively charged macromolecules during filtration. Since almost all plasma proteins bear net negative charges, this electrical hindrance plays a very important restrictive role, enhancing that of purely size hindrance. (For example, when neutral dextrans the size of plasma albumin are administered to experimental animals they are found to be 5 to 10 percent filterable, rather than the 0.02 percent of albumin.) Certain of the diseases that cause renal corpuscles to become "leaky" to protein do so by eliminating negative charges in the membranes.

It must be emphasized that the negative charges in the filtration membranes act as a hindrance only to macromolecules, not to mineral ions or low-molecular-weight organic solutes.

Finally, it should be noted that certain low-molecular-weight solutes that would otherwise be completely filterable are partially bound to large plasma proteins; the protein-bound moiety does not filter out of the glomerulus. The concentration of such a substance in Bowman's capsule will equal not the full plasma concentration but the plasma concentration of the substance not bound to protein. For example, 40 percent of the plasma calcium is protein-bound, and so the calcium concentration of the glomerular filtrate is 60 percent of that in plasma. (Such cases are the reason for use of the word "most" in the first sentence of this section.)

Direct Determinants of GFR

The rate of fluid movement, by filtration, in *any* of the body's capillaries is determined by the hydraulic permeability of the capillaries, their surface area, and the **net filtration pressure** (NFP) acting across them.

$$\text{Rate of filtration} = \text{hydraulic permeability} \times \text{surface area} \times \text{NFP}$$

Because it is difficult to estimate the area of a capillary bed, a parameter called the **filtration coefficient** (K_f) is used to denote the product of the hydraulic permeability and the area.[3] The NFP is the algebraic sum of the hydraulic pressures and the osmotic pressures due to protein—the oncotic (or colloid osmotic) pressures—on the two sides of the capillary wall. Applying this to the glomerular capillaries:

$$\text{NFP} = \underset{\text{forces inducing filtration}}{(P_{GC} + \Pi_{BC})} - \underset{\text{forces opposing filtration}}{(P_{BC} + \Pi_{GC})}$$

where P_{GC} = glomerular–capillary hydraulic pressure
Π_{BC} = oncotic pressure of fluid in Bowman's capsule
P_{BC} = hydraulic pressure in Bowman's capsule
Π_{GC} = oncotic pressure in glomerular–capillary plasma

Because there is virtually no protein in Bowman's capsule Π_{BC} may be taken as zero and not considered in our analysis (Fig. 2-1). Accordingly the overall equation for GFR becomes:

$$\text{GFR} = \underset{\substack{\text{(hydraulic permeability} \\ \times \text{ surface area)}}}{K_f} \times \underset{(P_{GC} - P_{BC} - \Pi_{GC})}{\text{NFP}}$$

The hydraulic pressures in glomerular capillaries and Bowman's capsule have not been directly measured in humans. However, several lines of indirect evidence suggest that the human values are probably similar to those for the dog, and these values are shown in Table 2-1 and Fig. 2-2 along with glomerular capillary oncotic pressure.

Note that the hydraulic pressure changes only very slightly along the glomeruli; this is because the very large total cross-sectional area of the glomeruli provides only small resistance to flow. Very importantly, note that the oncotic pressure in the glomerular capillaries changes quite a bit along the length of the glomeruli; since the filtrate is essentially protein-free, the filtration process removes water but not protein from the plasma, thereby increasing the protein concentration and, hence, the oncotic pressure of the unfiltered plasma remaining in the glomerular capillaries.[4] Mainly because of this large

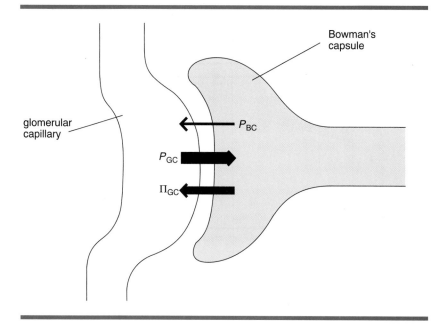

Fig. 2-1 Net filtration pressure in the renal corpuscle equals glomerular-capillary hydraulic pressure (P_{GC}) minus Bowman's capsule hydraulic pressure (P_{BC}) minus glomerular-capillary oncotic pressure (Π_{GC}).

increase in oncotic pressure the net filtration pressure decreases by a large amount from the beginning of the glomerular capillaries to the end, the average value being approximately 17 mmHg.[5] That this pressure suffices to cause the filtration of 180 L of fluid per day is attributable mainly to the fact that the hydraulic permeability and, hence, the K_f for glomerular capillaries, is several orders of magnitude greater than for nonrenal capillaries.

Table 2-1 Estimated Forces Involved in Glomerular Filtration in Humans

	mmHg	
Forces	Afferent end of glomerular capillary	Efferent end of glomerular capillary
1 Favoring filtration: Glomerular-capillary hydraulic pressure, P_{GC}	60	58
2 Opposing filtration: a Hydraulic pressure in Bowman's capsule, P_{BC}	15	15
b Oncotic pressure in glomerular capillary, Π_{GC}	21	33
3 Net filtration pressure (1 − 2)	24	10

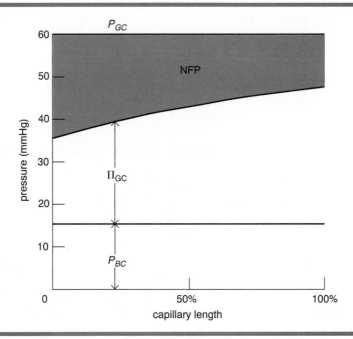

Fig. 2-2 Estimated forces involved in glomerular filtration in humans (these are the same values shown in Table 2-1). Net filtration pressure (NFP) = $P_{GC} - \Pi_{GC} - P_{BC}$.

The GFR is not fixed but may show marked fluctuations in differing physiological states and in disease. If all other factors remain constant, any change in K_f, P_{GC}, P_{BC}, or Π_{GC} will alter GFR. However, "all other factors" do not always remain constant, and so other simultaneous events may oppose the effect of the specific factor being analyzed. The phrase "tends to . . ." in the following discussion reflects this fact.

Table 2-2 presents a summary of the material to be described in the rest of this section. It provides, in essence, a checklist to go over when trying to understand how diseases or vasoactive chemical messengers and drugs change GFR. In this regard it should be noted that the major cause of decreased GFR in renal disease is not any change in these parameters within individual nephrons but rather simply a decrease in the number of functioning nephrons.

$\boldsymbol{K_f}$ Changes in K_f can be caused by glomerular disease and drugs, but this variable is also subject to normal physiological control by a variety of chemical messengers. The mechanism is not known, but one likely hypothesis is that these messengers cause contraction of glomerular mesangial cells, with a resulting decrease in glomerular surface area and, hence, K_f. This decrease in K_f will tend to lower GFR.[6]

Table 2-2 Summary of Direct GFR Determinants and Factors that Influence Them

Direct determinants of GFR: $GFR = K_f(P_{GC} - P_{BC} - \Pi_{GC})$	Major factors that tend to increase the magnitude of the direct determinant
K_f^*	(1) ↑ glomerular surface area (because of relaxation of glomerular mesangial cells) Result: ↑ GFR
P_{GC}^*	(1) ↑ renal arterial pressure (2) ↓ afferent-arteriolar resistance (afferent dilation) (3) ↑ efferent-arteriolar resistance (efferent constriction) Result: ↑ GFR
P_{BC}^*	(1) ↑ intratubular pressure because of obstruction of tubule or extrarenal urinary system Result: ↓ GFR
Π_{GC}^*	(1) ↑ systemic-plasma oncotic pressure (sets Π_{GC} at beginning of glomerular capillaries) (2) ↓ renal plasma flow (causes increased rise of Π_{GC} along glomerular capillaries) Result: ↓ GFR

*K_f = filtration coefficient; P_{GC} = glomerular-capillary hydraulic pressure; P_{BC} = Bowman's capsule hydraulic pressure; Π_{GC} = glomerular-capillary oncotic pressure. A reversal of all arrows in the table will cause a decrease in the magnitudes of K_f, P_{GC}, P_{BC}, and Π_{GC}.

P_{GC} P_{GC} reflects the interplay of renal arterial pressure, afferent-arteriolar resistance (R_A), and efferent-arteriolar resistance (R_E) (Fig. 2-3). First (not shown in Fig. 2-3), a change in renal arterial pressure will tend to cause a change in P_{GC} of the same direction (but for reasons described later in this chapter this change will be minimal). Second (Fig. 2-3B), at any given renal arterial pressure, an increase in R_A (due to afferent-arteriolar constriction) will tend to lower P_{GC}, simply by causing a greater loss of pressure between the renal arteries and glomerular capillaries. Conversely, a decrease in R_A (due to afferent-arteriolar dilation) will tend to raise P_{GC}. Third (Fig. 2-3C), and more difficult to visualize, is the fact that changes in R_E also tend to cause changes in P_{GC}, but *the changes are opposite to those caused by changes in R_A.* Thus, an increase in R_E (due to efferent-arteriolar constriction) tends to *elevate* P_{GC}. This occurs because the efferent arteriole lies beyond the glomerulus, so that efferent-arteriolar constriction tends to "dam back" the blood in the glomerular capillaries, raising P_{GC}. Similarly, a decrease in R_E (due to efferent-arteriolar dilation) tends to lower P_{GC}. It should also be clear that when R_A and R_E both change simultaneously in the *same* direction (i.e., both increase or decrease) they exert *opposing* effects on P_{GC} (Fig. 2-3D). When they change in *different* directions, they cause *additive* effects on P_{GC}.

Now recall the controls of RBF and see how totally different the story is for this parameter; for RBF, changes in R_A and R_E in the *same* direction

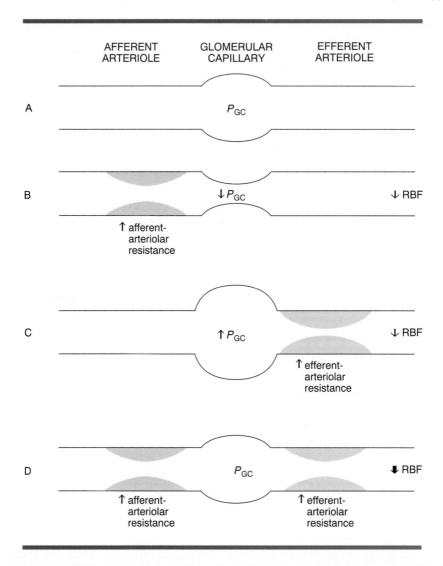

Fig. 2-3 Effects of afferent- and/or efferent-arteriolar constriction on glomerular-capillary pressure (P_{GC}) and renal blood flow (RBF). The RBF changes reflect changes in *total* renal arteriolar resistance, the location of the change being irrelevant. In contrast, the changes in P_{GC} reflect in which set of arterioles the altered resistance occurs. Pure afferent constriction (*B*) lowers both P_{GC} and RBF, whereas pure efferent constriction (*C*) raises P_{GC} and lowers RBF. Simultaneous constriction of both afferent and efferent arterioles (*D*) has counteracting effects on P_{GC} but additive effects on RBF; the effect on P_{GC} may be a small increase, small decrease, or no change. Vasodilation of only one set of arterioles would have effects on P_{GC} and RBF opposite to those shown in parts *B* and *C*. Vasodilation of both sets would cause little or no change in P_{GC}, the same result as constriction of both sets, but would cause a large increase in RBF. Constriction of one set of arterioles and dilation of the other would have maximal effects on P_{GC} but little effect on RBF.

cause *additive* effects on RBF, whereas changes in *different* directions cause *opposing* effects.

P_{BC} Changes in this variable generally are of very minor *physiological* importance. The major *pathological* cause of increased hydraulic pressure in Bowman's capsule is obstruction anywhere along the tubule or in the external portions of the urinary system (e.g., the ureter). The effect of such an occlusion is to increase the tubular pressure everywhere proximal to the occlusion, all the way back to Bowman's capsule. The result is to decrease GFR.

Π_{GC} Oncotic pressure in the plasma at the very beginning of the glomerular capillaries is, of course, simply the oncotic pressure of systemic arterial plasma. Accordingly, a decrease in arterial plasma protein concentration, as occurs, for example, in liver disease, will lower arterial oncotic pressure and tend to increase GFR, whereas increased arterial oncotic pressure will tend to reduce GFR.

But now recall (Table 2-1 and Fig. 2-2) that Π_{GC} is identical to arterial oncotic pressure only at the very beginning of the glomerular capillaries; Π_{GC} then progressively increases along the glomerular capillaries as protein-free fluid filters out of the capillary, concentrating the protein left behind. This means that net filtration pressure and, hence, filtration, progressively decrease along the capillary length. Accordingly, *anything that causes a steeper rise in* Π_{GC} *will tend to lower average net filtration pressure and hence GFR.*

This tends to occur when renal plasma flow (RPF) is low. It shouldn't be hard to visualize that the filtration of a given volume of fluid from a small total volume of plasma flowing through the glomeruli will cause the protein left behind to become more concentrated than if the total volume of plasma were large. In other words, the presence of a low RPF, all other factors remaining constant, will cause the Π_{GC} to rise more steeply and reach a final value at the end of the glomerular capillaries which is higher than normal.[7] This increase in average Π_{GC} along the capillaries lowers average net filtration pressure and, hence, GFR. Conversely, a high RPF, all other factors remaining constant, will cause Π_{GC} to rise less steeply and reach a final value at the end of the capillaries that is less than normal, which will increase the GFR.[8]

Another way of thinking about this is in terms of filtration fraction—the ratio GFR/RPF. The increase in Π_{GC} along the glomerular capillaries is directly proportional to the filtration fraction; i.e., the more of a given RPF that is filtered the higher the rise in Π_{GC}. Therefore, if you know that filtration fraction has changed, you can be certain that there has been a greater or lesser increase in Π_{GC} and that this has played a role in altering GFR.

MEAN ARTERIAL PRESSURE AND AUTOREGULATION

Look again at Equation 2-1. This equation predicts that if the pressure gradient is increased by 50 percent, blood flow will increase 50 percent. In the kidney, however, this does not occur because the renal circulation manifests quite markedly the phenomenon of **autoregulation:** The RBF remains relatively constant in response to changes in mean renal arterial pressure in the range between approximately 85 and 200 mmHg (Fig. 2-4).

For example, if one isolates a kidney experimentally and perfuses it with blood by means of a pump, one can demonstrate that a 50 percent increase in renal arterial pressure (say, from 100 mmHg to 150 mmHg) produces less than a 10 percent increase in RBF. As can be deduced from Equation 2-1, there is only one possible explanation for this: Resistance in the kidney must also have increased as arterial pressure was increased. The smooth muscle of the renal arterioles contracted to a greater degree, thereby decreasing the radii of the arterioles and, hence, increasing arteriolar resistance. Therefore, RBF remained relatively unchanged despite the increased arterial pressure.

This entire discussion applies not only to RBF but also to GFR, which also shows only small changes in response to large changes in arterial pressure. The main reason that GFR, as well as RBF, is autoregulated is that the *afferent* arterioles are the major site of autoregulatory resistance changes in response to arterial pressure changes. Therefore, glomerular-capillary pressure and net filtration pressure remain relatively unchanged. In other words, a *rise* in renal arterial pressure triggers *increased* afferent-arteriolar constriction, thereby increasing the pressure drop between the arteries and glomerular capillaries and preventing the transmission of the increased arterial pressure to the glomerular capillaries.

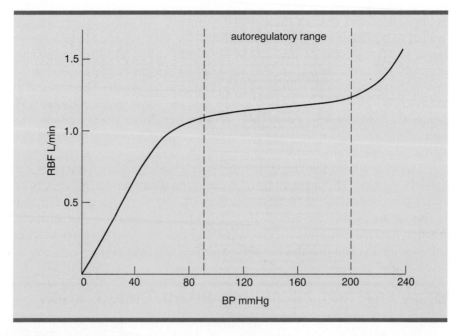

Fig. 2-4 Autoregulation of renal blood flow (RBF). A similar pattern holds for glomerular filtration rate.

By what mechanism does an increase in renal arterial pressure elicit enhanced contraction of the smooth muscle of the afferent arterioles? One thing is certain: The mechanism is completely intrarenal since it can be elicited in an isolated kidney perfused in vitro. Two intrarenal mechanisms are presently thought to be responsible for autoregulation: (1) a **myogenic mechanism;** and (2) **tubuloglomerular feedback.**

The myogenic mechanism is similar to that found in other (nonrenal) autoregulating vascular beds: Vascular smooth muscle contracts in response to increased *stretch*. Accordingly, an increased intra-arteriolar pressure distends the arteriolar wall, i.e., increases its passive tension, and the inherent response of the smooth muscle in the wall is to contract, thereby increasing the resistance offered by the vessel.

Compared to the myogenic mechanism, tubuloglomerular feedback is a more complex process, which primarily regulates GFR, with changes in RBF as a secondary consequence. The basic pathway is illustrated in Fig. 2-5. (As preparation for this discussion, the reader should review, if necessary, the anatomy of the juxtaglomerular apparatus (JGA) in Chapter 1.) Increased arterial pressure tends to raise both glomerular-capillary pressure (P_{GC}) and RBF. The increase in P_{GC} raises GFR and, hence, the rate of fluid flow through the proximal tubule and loop of Henle, including the macula densa—the plaque of cells near the end of the thick ascending limb of Henle's loop. As a result of the increased flow through the macula densa (see below and Fig. 2-5 for the mechanism by which flow is "detected"), a vasoconstrictor chemical is generated in the JGA. This vasoconstrictor stimulates the smooth muscle of the adjacent afferent arterioles; the result is an increased afferent-arteriolar resistance, which decreases P_{GC} and, hence, GFR,[9] as well as RBF back toward their original values. In other words, the arteriolar constriction greatly dampens the increases in GFR and RBF that would otherwise have been caused by the elevated renal arterial pressure.

Now let us back up and discuss more specifically some of the mechanisms that underlie tubuloglomerular feedback. First, how does the macula densa "detect" changes in rate of fluid flow? The answer is as follows (Fig. 2-5): Because the thick ascending limb of Henle's loop actively reabsorbs sodium and chloride but not water (as will be described in detail in Chapter 6), the luminal concentrations of the two ions are always lower than those of plasma, and there is a direct relationship between the luminal flow rate and the concentrations of the ions—i.e., the higher the flow rate the higher the sodium chloride concentrations. These increased concentrations in turn cause the macula densa to reabsorb more sodium and chloride,[10] and it is this increased reabsorption that somehow causes increased production of the vasoconstrictor that acts on the afferent arterioles.

What is the identity of the vasoconstrictor in this system? **Adenosine**, which constricts afferent arterioles, in contrast to its vasodilator effects on other vascular beds in the body, is the most important mediator.[11]

The examples used to illustrate the myogenic and tubuloglomerular mechanisms for autoregulation used an *increase* in renal arterial pressure as the

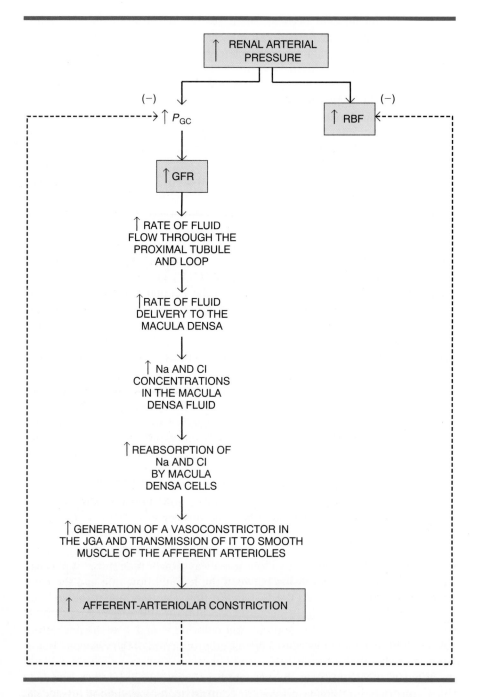

Fig. 2-5 Tubuloglomerular feedback contribution to autoregulation. The major vaso-constrictor in this pathway is adenosine.

initial event. *Decreases* in arterial pressure within the autoregulatory range are also offset by autoregulation: Decreased stretch of afferent-arteriolar smooth muscle causes relaxation, i.e., less contraction, and decreased flow through the macula densa causes less adenosine to be produced by the JGA (and possibly increased production of a vasodilator as well—see note 11).

What is the adaptive value of autoregulation? First, as in any other autoregulating organ, it helps prevent major blood-flow changes in the face of arterial-pressure fluctuations. But it also serves a second role in the kidney, namely the blunting of the large changes in solute and water excretion that would *otherwise* occur because of large changes in GFR whenever arterial pressure changed. This is the adaptive value of GFR autoregulation. Recall that the normal net filtration pressure in the glomeruli is only about 17 mmHg. Accordingly, even relatively minor changes in arterial pressure could cause marked changes in glomerular-capillary pressure, GFR, and solute and water excretion, were the changes not effectively blunted by automatic changes in afferent-arteriolar tonus.

In this regard, it should be emphasized that although we introduced tubuloglomerular feedback in the context of autoregulation, this feedback process is important in situations characterized not by changes in arterial pressure but rather by disease-induced or drug-induced blockade of fluid reabsorption in the proximal tubule.[12] Under such conditions, the resulting increase in macula densa flow triggers, via the usual sequence of events, a decrease in GFR and thereby limits the urinary loss of salt and water resulting from the defect in reabsorption. Note that in these cases, tubuloglomerular feedback actually causes GFR to go *down*, whereas during autoregulatory responses, it keeps GFR from changing.

Having pointed out the value of autoregulation, we must now emphasize three facts: (1) Even within the autoregulatory range autoregulation is not perfect; RBF and GFR *do change* when renal arterial pressure is changed, but much less than they would if autoregulation did not exist (Fig. 2-4). (2) Autoregulation is virtually absent at mean arterial pressures below 70 mmHg and, therefore, cannot blunt GRF and RBF changes below this value, a point of great importance for renal function during severe systemic hypotension. (3) Despite autoregulation, RBF and GFR (to a lesser extent) *can be altered considerably*, even when the arterial pressure is within the autoregulatory range, by neuroendocrine factors—particularly the sympathetic nervous system and angiotensin II—to be described in the next two sections.

Because of this last fact, we set up artificial experimental conditions in the above discussion of autoregulation in which renal blood pressure was changed without altering blood pressure elsewhere in the body (an analogue of this in a person would be an obstruction in a renal artery). Such experimental conditions are necessary to demonstrate "pure" autoregulation because when the systemic arterial pressure decreases everywhere in the *intact* organism, neuroendocrine reflexes are brought into play that mask the occurrence of autoregulation.

RENAL SYMPATHETIC NERVES

The afferent and efferent arterioles are richly supplied with **sympathetic neu-rons**, which release norepinephrine. This neurotransmitter acts on both the afferent and efferent arterioles, via α-adrenergic receptors, to cause constriction of both sets of arterioles (Fig. 2-6). Vascular resistance therefore increases in both sets, causing a decrease in RBF that is proportional to the increase in total resistance. Circulating **epinephrine** also causes renal vasoconstriction via α-adrenergic receptors,[13] but for simplicity and because the renal nerves are the more potent input, we will usually mention only the latter, tacitly including

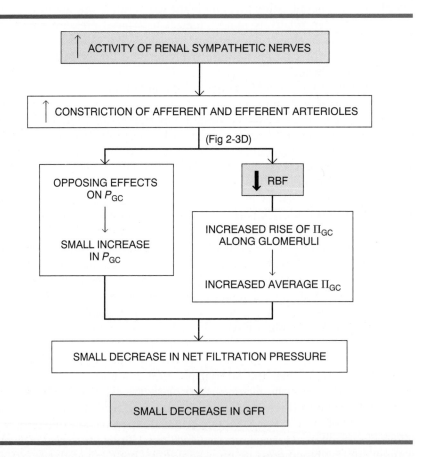

Fig. 2-6 Effects of increased activity of the renal sympathetic nerves on renal blood flow (RBF) and glomerular filtration rate (GFR). The changes shown in this figure are for a moderate-to-large increase in renal sympathetic-nerve activity. Commonly, a relatively small increase in nerve activity may cause no change at all in GFR (despite a decreased RBF) because it produces identical changes in P_{GC} and Π_{GC}. As described in the text, the effects of angiotensin II on the renal arterioles and, hence, on RBF and GFR are qualitatively similar to those exerted by the sympathetic nerves.

epinephrine as well. In a resting, unstressed person, the sympathetic-nerve activity to the kidneys is too low to influence renal hemodynamics, but a reflexly induced increase in sympathetic outflow will cause renal arteriolar constriction and reduce RBF.

What does the increased sympathetic activity do to GFR (Fig. 2-6)? To answer this question, we apply the approach given in Table 2-2. (1) It is uncertain whether the renal nerves alter K_f. (2) The nerves produce opposing changes in P_{GC} (as in Fig. 2-3D); the afferent-arteriolar constriction *decreases* P_{GC}, whereas the *efferent*-arteriolar constriction does just the opposite. The net effect observed experimentally is a small rise in P_{GC}, which tends to *increase* GFR. (3) The renal nerves produce no significant effect on P_{BC}. (4) Because of the decrease in RBF and, hence, RPF caused by the nerves, there is a steeper rise in Π_{GC} along the glomerular capillaries, which tends to *reduce* GFR.

Clearly we have here opposing effects on GFR. The rise in Π_{GC} is generally the same as or slightly greater than the rise in P_{GC}, and so net filtration pressure remains constant or decreases slightly. Therefore, the GFR remains unchanged or goes down slightly, not nearly as much as RBF does (Fig. 2-6). These are the effects seen when the activity of the renal sympathetic nerves is only moderately increased. With larger increases the fall in GFR becomes more pronounced but is still always much less than the fall in RBF. Because increased activity of the renal nerves causes RBF and, hence, RPF to go down more than GFR, it produces an increase in filtration fraction. We shall make use of this fact, which should help you remember that the renal nerves cause a greater rise in Π_{GC} along the glomeruli, in Chapter 7 when we discuss fluid reabsorption.

Finally, it should be noted that this section has dealt only with the *direct* effects of the sympathetic nerves and circulating epinephrine on renal arterioles. As we shall see below, the sympathetic nerves stimulate renin secretion and the resulting increase in angiotensin II also causes renal arteriolar constriction very much like the direct effects of the nerves. In other words, in addition to their direct arteriolar action, the sympathetic nerves indirectly constrict renal arterioles via angiotensin II.

Reflexes Involving the Renal Sympathetic Nerves

One of the major reflexes influencing renal sympathetic nerves is the classic arterial-baroreceptor reflex: As illustrated for hemorrhage in Fig. 2-7, a decrease in pressure within the carotid sinuses and aortic arch baroreceptors reflexly elicits increased activity of the sympathetic nerves to the kidneys. What is the adaptive value of these reflexes? For one thing, it is simply a component of the rapid general homeostatic regulation of arterial pressure. The renal vasoconstriction contributes to a rise in total peripheral resistance (TPR), which helps rapidly to restore the arterial blood pressure toward normal (Fig. 2-7). But there is a second, less obvious, way in which renal vasoconstriction helps raise arterial pressure, namely by reducing the excretion of sodium and water and thereby retaining more fluid in the body. Renal vasoconstriction achieves a reduction in salt and water excretion both by lowering GFR (and,

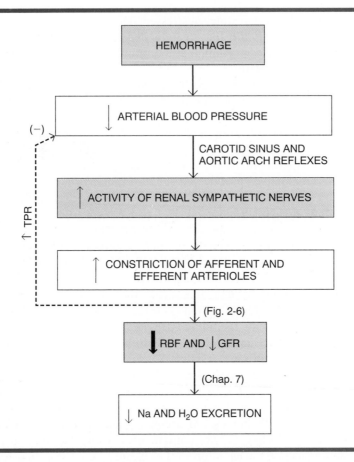

Fig. 2-7 Pathway by which arterial hypotension causes, via arterial baroreceptors, reflex vasoconstriction mediated by the renal sympathetic nerves (epinephrine, released from the adrenal medulla, enhances the renal vasoconstriction). Decreases in venous and cardiac pressures also elicit the same response via baroreceptors in these structures. This figure shows only the *direct* effects of the renal sympathetic nerves on the arterioles; in addition, as summarized in the text and Figs. 2-9 and 2-10, these nerves also stimulate renin secretion, and the resulting increase in angiotensin II also constricts the renal arterioles.

hence, the filtered load of these substances) and, as we shall see in Chapter 7, by increasing tubular reabsorption of these substances.

The same type of sympathetically mediated vasoconstriction can be reflexly triggered by baroreceptors in the veins and cardiac chambers. Indeed, input from these baroreceptors probably has greater reflex sympathetic effects on the renal circulation than does input from the arterial baroreceptors. Input from the peripheral chemoreceptors (responding to hypoxia or reduced plasma pH) or from higher brain centers (e.g., during heavy exercise or emotional situations) can also trigger increased sympathetic outflow to the kidneys.

ANGIOTENSIN II

A second major regulator of the renal circulation is the renin-angiotensin system. (At this point, the student should review the basic biochemistry of this hormonal system given in Chapter 1.) Angiotensin II, which functions in the kidneys as both a hormone and a paracrine agent, is a very powerful vasoconstrictor; it acts on both the afferent and efferent arterioles to raise renal vascular resistance and, thereby, reduce RBF.[14]

What about GFR? The effects of angiotensin II on the determinants of net filtration pressure are qualitatively similar to those just described for the sympathetic nerves (Fig. 2-6): The combined afferent and efferent constriction causes a rise in P_{GC}, whereas the decrease in RPF causes an increase in the average Π_{GC}. But, in addition, angiotensin II definitely reduces K_f, presumably by an action on the glomerular mesangial cells. The GFR-decreasing effects of the reduced K_f and the elevated Π_{GC} equal or exceed the GFR-increasing effect of the elevated P_{GC}, and so the GFR remains unchanged or goes down, but only a small amount. Again, similar to the renal sympathetic nerves, higher concentrations of angiotensin II cause larger falls in GFR, but still not as much as the decrease in RPF. Therefore, filtration fraction always increases.

As described in Chapter 1, the plasma and local intrarenal concentrations of angiotensin II are increased when the kidneys are stimulated to secrete more renin. Accordingly, angiotensin-induced renal hemodynamic changes can be expected whenever renin secretion is signficantly elevated.

Control of Renin Secretion

Renin secretion is controlled by four major types of inputs, which are strongly interrelated: (1) input from intrarenal baroreceptors, (2) input from the macula densa, (3) a β-adrenergic mechanism mediated by the renal sympathetic nerves and epinephrine, and (4) angiotensin II itself. There are many inputs other than these four that are capable of altering renin release, but under most physiological circumstances they are of lesser importance.[15] (One of these other inputs—the inhibition caused by the hormone called atrial natriuretic factor—is described in Chapter 7.)

Intrarenal Baroreceptors The renin-secreting granular cells of the juxtaglomerular apparatus themselves act as **intrarenal baroreceptors**, monitoring the pressure or vascular volume within the afferent arterioles and varying their secretion of renin *inversely* with these parameters. Accordingly, whenever arterial pressure decreases, renin release will be stimulated by the intrarenal baroreceptors (Fig. 2-8). Conversely, an increased arterial pressure will inhibit renin release.

Macula Densa Earlier in this chapter, we described how the macula densa is involved in tubuloglomerular feedback. Now we describe another completely distinct function for the macula densa—control of renin secretion.

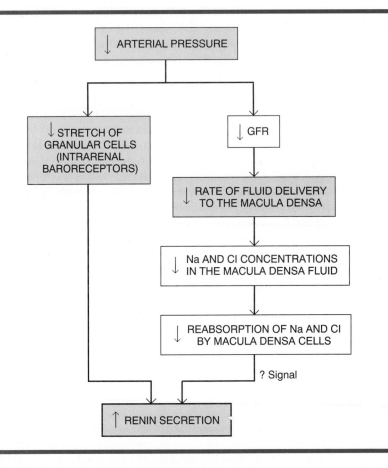

Fig. 2-8   A decrease in arterial blood pressure stimulates renin secretion by both the intrarenal baroreceptors and macula densa receptors.

In discussing tubuloglomerular feedback, we pointed out that an increased flow to the macula densa is accompanied by increased sodium and chloride concentrations in the macula densa lumen and, hence, increased sodium chloride reabsorption by the macula densa cells. We stated that this increased reabsorption somehow generates the signal for *increased* production of the vasoconstrictor agent—adenosine—that mediates tubuloglomerular feedback. Now we point out that this same signal, increased sodium chloride reabsorption by the macula densa, elicits *inhibition* of renin release; the pathway by which this occurs is still not clear.[16] Conversely, when flow and, hence, sodium and chloride concentrations in the macula densa are low, renin secretion is stimulated.

Thus, the macula densa mechanism causes increased renin secretion when there is a decrease in GFR and/or an increase in fluid reabsorption by the proximal tubule, since these are the two events that cause decreased macula densa flow. When a decrease in arterial blood pressure is the cause of a decreased GFR (remember that autoregulation does not completely prevent changes in GFR induced by altered blood pressure), the macula densa and intrarenal baroreceptors "cooperate," i.e., they both stimulate renin secretion (Fig. 2-8). Conversely, when arterial pressure increases, both the intrarenal baroreceptor and the macula densa signal for decreased renin secretion.

Renal Sympathetic Nerves   Sympathetic neurons end in the immediate vicinity of the granular cells, and these neurons exert a *direct* stimulatory effect on renin secretion via β_1-adrenergic receptors on the granular cells (Fig. 2-9). This is the major mechanism by which increased activity of the renal nerves stimulates renin secretion. Conversely, a decrease in sympathetic-nerve activity results in decreased renin secretion.

    There is also an *indirect* way that the renal nerves can stimulate renin release, namely by reducing the flow to the macula densa. As described earlier in this chapter, increased activity of the renal nerves can lower the GFR, and

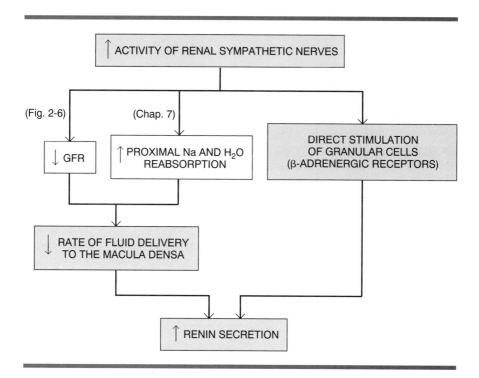

Fig. 2-9 The renal sympathetic nerves stimulate renin secretion by a direct effect on the granular cells (mediated by β_1-adrenergic receptors) and by causing a decrease in flow to the macula densa. The direct effect is the most important of these two pathways. The mechanisms by which increased sympathetic activity enhances sodium and water reabsorption by the proximal tubule are described in Chapter 7.

we shall see in Chapter 7 that it can also increase proximal-tubular fluid reabsorption. The net effect will be to lower fluid delivery to the macula densa, which will stimulate renin release (Fig. 2-9).[17]

Thus, in the many situations in which there is a reflex increase in the activity of the renal sympathetic nerves (see previous section) renin secretion will usually also be increased. Figure 2-10 summarizes the integrated responses of the two intrarenal receptor mechanisms and the renal nerves in response to hemorrhage.

Angiotensin II   Angiotensin II exerts a direct inhibitory effect on renin secretion by the granular cells. This is an example of a negative feedback in which a hormone inhibits the secretion of its own stimulating substance, analogous to the inhibition of ACTH secretion by cortisol or to inhibition of TSH secretion by thyroxine. By this mechanism, angiotensin II exerts a dampening effect on its own rate of production.

Adaptive Value of Increased Renin Release   Because I have presented the control of renin secretion in the context of the regulation of *renal* hemodynamics the reader might easily gain the (incorrect) impression that the sole or major function of the renin-angiotensin system is to regulate these

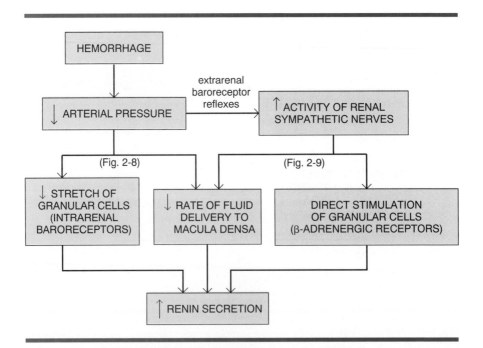

Fig. 2-10 Hemorrhage causes increased renin release by all three of the inputs controlling secretion of this hormone. This figure contains no new information but is merely an amalgamation of Figs. 2-8 and 2-9.

hemodynamics. In fact, angiotensin II has other, more important, actions. First, angiotensin II not only constricts renal arterioles but arterioles in most organs and tissues; accordingly, an increased plasma angiotensin II concentration will increase total peripheral resistance and raise arterial blood pressure. Second, by several direct and indirect mechanisms to be described in Chapter 7, angiotensin II causes the tubular reabsorption of sodium to increase, which (along with the small decrease in GFR that angiotensin II produces) causes retention of sodium in the body. Thus the adaptive value of increased renin release—and hence an increased plasma angiotensin II concentration—in response to hemorrhage or other situations in which arterial pressure is low is the same as that described earlier for increased activity of the renal sympathetic nerves: (1) It increases total peripheral resistance and thereby raises arterial blood pressure; and (2) it helps retain sodium in the body. We'll return to these phenomena in Chapter 7 when we describe the reflexes that control total-body sodium.

PROSTAGLANDINS

Several of the renally produced prostaglandins, notably **PGE$_2$** and **PGI$_2$**, are vasodilators. In the normal unstressed state they are produced in concentrations too low to influence the renal arterioles. In contrast, increased activity of the renal nerves or increased angiotensin II stimulates the kidneys to synthesize and release large amounts of these vasodilator prostaglandins, which then act locally on both afferent and efferent arterioles (as well as on glomerular mesangial cells). The end result is that much of the vasoconstrictor actions of norepinephrine and angiotensin II are counteracted by the vasodilator actions of the prostaglandins, and the renal resistance changes much less than would otherwise have occurred (Fig. 2-11).[18] The adaptive value of such opposing inputs is to strike a balance between, on the one hand, the requirement for an increased total peripheral resistance to maintain systemic arterial pressure (for the "benefit" of the heart and brain) and, on the other hand, the likelihood of renal damage if renal vasoconstriction were too severe.[19]

In summary, if we return once more to our example of hypotension due to hemorrhage, we see that three major factors are reducing renal blood flow (and, to a lesser extent, GFR)—the decreased blood pressure per se, the renal sympathetic nerves, and angiotensin II. Simultaneously, two factors are minimizing the reduction—autoregulation and the vasodilator prostaglandins, whose release is stimulated by the renal nerves and angiotensin II. The net result is usually a modest increase in renal vascular resistance, leading to a modest decrease in RBF (and an even smaller decrease in GFR).

OTHER FACTORS

I have presented only those factors presently thought to be most important in the reflex control of RBF and GFR. The renal vasculature is, however, sensitive to many other chemical messengers. Indeed, the renal arterioles have

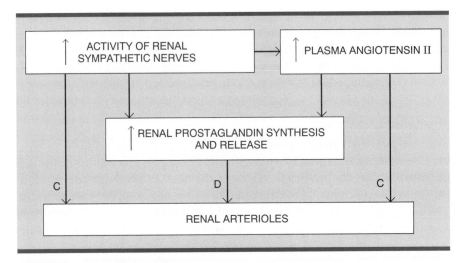

Fig. 2-11 "Dampening" effect of prostaglandins on renal vasoconstriction induced by the renal nerves or angiotensin II. C = constriction; D = dilation.

receptors for more than 25 vasoactive neurotransmitters, hormones, and paracrine agents, and there are more than 20 vasoactive substances produced by cells of the renal corpuscles alone!

The importance of all these potential messengers with regard to the renal circulation is, in many cases, still unclear. Some of them (for example, endothelium-derived relaxing factor) are almost certainly involved in normal physiological control. Others—particularly those intrarenal paracrine agents that cause vasoconstriction—may turn out to have minor physiological roles but be very important in the generation of renal disease. Still others may have no role at all. The names and overall actions—whether vasodilator or vasoconstrictor—of some of these additional messengers are given *for reference* in Table 2-3 (for further information on these see the Suggested Readings), along with the well-known neuroendocrine messengers described in this chapter. You will surely be encountering many others, as well as a host of vasoactive drugs, in the future.

For review, let me emphasize again that once you know the effects of a messenger (or drug) on the renal arterioles you should be able to deduce how the messenger influences RBF and GFR.

1. Most vasoactive agents tend to exert the same effect—vasoconstrictor or vasodilator—on both sets of arterioles, although one effect may be larger than the other. As we saw for both angiotensin II and norepinephrine, such a vasoconstrictor will definitely lower RBF. It may also lower GFR, but to a much smaller extent.
2. The logic is the same but in the opposite direction for a vasodilator of both sets of arterioles. It will definitely raise RBF and may also raise GFR, but to a much smaller extent.

Table 2-3 Some Chemical Messengers that Influence the Renal Vasculature

VASOCONSTRICTORS[†]

Name (category*)	Comment
Norepinephrine and epinephrine (NT; H)	See text for detailed description
Angiotensin II (H, P)	See text for detailed description
Antidiuretic hormone (H) (ADH, vasopressin)	Only effective at very high plasma concentrations
Adenosine (P)	Is the major mediator in tubuloglomerular feedback Causes afferent constriction but efferent dilation
Thromboxane A_2 (TXA$_2$) (P)	May cause vasoconstriction in renal diseases
Leukotrienes (P)	May cause vasoconstriction in renal diseases
Endothelin (P)	May cause vasoconstriction in renal diseases

VASODILATORS[†]

PGE$_2$ and PGI$_2$ (prostacyclin) (P)	See text for detailed description
Atrial natriuretic factor (ANF) (H)	See Chapter 8 for detailed description Causes afferent dilation but efferent constriction
Endothelium-derived relaxing factor (EDRF, nitric oxide) (P)	Normally released tonically from vascular endothelial cells and contributes importantly to maintaining renal arterioles more dilated than they otherwise would be
Dopamine (NT)	Function presently uncertain
Bradykinin (P)	Function presently uncertain

*N = neurotransmitter; H = hormone; P = paracrine (or autocrine) agent.

†This describes the major effect of the messenger. Some of them act on both the afferent and efferent arterioles, whereas others are more specific for one or the other. In still other cases (adenosine and atrial natriuretic factor) a single agent may have opposite actions on the two sets of arterioles. Many of these messengers also affect K_f.

3. The overall effects of an agent that constricts one set of arterioles and dilates the other are also predictable. Since the two resistance changes oppose each other, the RBF will generally change only a small amount, if at all, depending on whether one of the effects is greater than the other (i.e., depending on whether *total* resistance changes). In contrast, the GFR changes will be very large because the effects on the two sets of arterioles are both causing P_{GC} to change in the same direction. Thus, for example, you should be able to deduce from the information given in Table 2-3 that atrial natriuretic factor has relatively little effect on RBF but causes a substantial increase in GFR.

4. Finally, if the K_f is known to be altered, you can factor this into the analysis: A decrease in K_f will favor a reduction in GFR, but will have no effect on RBF.

Study questions: 5 to 16

NOTES

[1]Actually, for two reasons related to the presence of protein in plasma but not in glomerular filtrate, the concentrations of completely filterable solutes in Bowman's capsule are not *exactly* the same as in plasma: (1) Solutes are, of course, dissolved in water, not protein, and the presence of the plasma proteins causes the plasma water to occupy only 95 percent of the total plasma volume. (2) The plasma proteins cause a Donnan equilibrium to exist between these fluids and this affects the concentrations of ions. Both these effects are small, however, and may be ignored for simplicity.

[2]It is likely that the endothelial cells, the basement membrane, and the slit diaphragms all play roles, depending upon the electrical charge on the macromolecules being filtered. (See Dworkin and Brenner in Suggested Readings.)

[3]The filtration process that occurs in the renal corpuscle is often called *ultrafiltration* to denote the fact that proteins are excluded. Accordingly K_f is often called the ultrafiltration coefficient.

[4]For physiochemical reasons we will not discuss, the relationship between oncotic pressure and plasma protein concentration is not linear. Oncotic pressure increases proportionally more than plasma protein concentration at protein concentrations greater than those of normal plasma.

[5]It should be noted that in several species of experimental animals, glomerular-capillary hydraulic pressure normally is lower than the value observed in dogs. Therefore, net filtration pressure is also lower and may actually become zero at some point along the glomerular capillary, a phenomenon known as *filtration pressure equilibrium.* This situation may also occur in human beings when glomerular-capillary pressure is unusually low, as, for example following a severe hemorrhage. Why the existence of filtration pressure equilibrium is important is given in notes 6–8. (See Dworkin and Brenner; and Maddox, Deen, and Brenner, in Suggested Readings.)

[6]The basic equation relating K_f and GFR predicts that any decrease in K_f should definitely cause a directly proportional decrease in GFR. However, this prediction does not apply to GFR under conditions in which glomerular filtration pressure equilibrium (see previous note) occurs well before the end of the glomerular capillaries. Under this condition, filtration, although reduced proportionally to K_f at every locus along the length of the capillary, will continue beyond the point in the capillary at which filtration pressure equilibrium previously had occurred. In this way, the total volume filtered along the entire length of capillary may change little, if at all. Because, as stated in note 5, filtration pressure equilibrium is probably not usual in human beings, changes in K_f should be taken into account. (See Dworkin and Brenner; and Maddox, Deen, and Brenner, in Suggested Readings.)

[7]Indeed, when renal plasma flow is very low, the Π_{GC} may become high enough before the end of the capillaries to equal the hydraulic pressure difference across the capillaries, at which point filtration ceases.

[8]Thus, changes in Π_{GC} constitute an automatic link between RPF and GFR, an increase or decrease in RPF tending to cause a change of similar direction in GFR. In those

animal species in which filtration pressure equilibrium normally occurs at some point along the glomerular capillaries (see above, note 5), the link is very tight. The reason is that the steeper rise in Π_{GC} resulting from the lower RPF causes the Π_{GC} to become equal to the hydraulic pressure difference across the glomerular capillaries at an earlier point than usual along the length of the capillaries. Accordingly, filtration ceases at this earlier point. Note that in these species the final Π_{GC} at the end of the glomerular capillaries is always equal to the hydraulic pressure and, therefore, is "set" by this latter pressure. In humans, however, the link between RPF and GFR is normally much less tight. (See Suggested Readings given in note 5.)

[9]A decrease in P_{GC} may not be the only reason that GFR decreases. Some evidence suggests that the vasoconstrictor released by the JGA acts not only on the afferent arterioles but on the glomerular mesangial cells as well. As described earlier, contraction of these mesangial cells would reduce the surface area of the glomeruli, thereby decreasing the filtration coefficient (K_f). (See Schnermann and Briggs in Suggested Readings.)

[10]The crucial luminal concentration determining the activity of the cotransporter that reabsorbs sodium and chloride in the macula densa (the same as that in the thick ascending loop, described in Chapter 6) is that of the chloride ion. This is because the sodium sites on the cotransporter are fully saturated at very low luminal sodium concentrations, whereas the chloride sites on the cotransporter show increased saturation over the entire range of physiological luminal chloride concentrations.

[11]It is not clear which cells of the JGA (or possibly even cells of the thick ascending limb of Henle's loop) produce the adenosine. Angiotensin II and several prostaglandins may play permissive roles in tubuloglomerular feedback but are definitely not the primary mediators of this process. Recent evidence also suggests that endothelium-derived relaxing factor (EDRF, nitric oxide), a vasodilator, may also play an important role; in this scenario, the JGA would tonically produce EDRF at a rate inversely proportional to macula densa flow rate. (See Schnermann and Briggs, and Jackson in Suggested Readings.)

[12]You might logically conclude that drugs that block fluid reabsorption in Henle's loop would also trigger tubuloglomerular feedback effects similar to those occurring with proximal-tubular blockade. However, loop-acting drugs block sodium and chloride reabsorption by the macula densa and so actually eliminate the feedback signal. (See Schnermann and Briggs in Suggested Readings.)

[13]There are also some β-adrenergic receptors on renal arteriolar smooth muscle, but so few in comparison to the α-adrenergic receptors that epinephrine causes only vasoconstriction in the kidneys.

[14]The action on the efferent arterioles is much greater than on the afferent. Indeed, there is a real question as to whether angiotensin II exerts any effect at all on afferent arterioles, but the evidence presently favors the conclusion that this hormone normally does have some afferent effect. (See Navar and Stein in Suggested Readings.)

[15]These include increases in the plasma concentrations of ADH, potassium, and calcium, all of which can inhibit renin release. In contrast, an increase in plasma hydrogen-

ion concentration stimulates renin release. The physiological significance of all these inputs is mainly that they provide additional loops in the feedback mechanisms integrating the metabolism of sodium with that of water and the other ions. Atrial natriuretic factor also inhibits renin release, the significance of which is discussed in Chapter 8.

Also of significance for renin release are the many renal paracrine agents. In particular, several of the prostaglandins produced within the kidneys, notably PGE_2 and PGI_2, can stimulate renin secretion, and these prostaglandins act as mediators or modulators of certain of the other inputs. Present evidence suggests that β-adrenergic control over renin secretion is independent of prostaglandins but that the prostaglandins function as important mediators in the macula densa pathway mechanism and possibly also in the intrarenal-baroreceptor mechanism. (See Schnermann and Briggs, in Suggested Readings.) Another renal paracrine agent that plays at least some role in the macula densa pathway is adenosine, which can inhibit renin release (see note 16). Still other renal paracrine agents that can influence renin release are bradykinin, endothelium-derived relaxing factor, transforming growth factor-beta, and endothelin.

The large number of inputs that alter renin release act on the granular cells by a variety of signal-transduction mechanisms: (1) They influence cytosolic calcium concentration, but in this regard the granular cells are unusual secretory cells—renin secretion is inversely correlated with cytosolic calcium concentration; (2) they influence cAMP, renin release being directly correlated with cytosolic cAMP. (See Schnermann and Briggs in Suggested Readings.)

[16]Adenosine, the vasoconstrictor that mediates most or all of tubuloglomerular feedback, is also known to be an inhibitor of renin release. It is likely, therefore, that this substance simultaneously causes the vasoconstriction of tubuloglomerular feedback and inhibits renin release. However, present evidence indicates that adenosine is not the sole mediator of macula-densa triggered inhibition of renin release and that other substances must be involved. (See Schnermann and Briggs, and Jackson in Suggested Readings.)

[17]This section has described how the renal sympathetic nerves stimulate renin secretion. In fact, the reverse causal interaction also exists, in that angiotensin II enhances the release of norepinephrine from renal sympathetic nerve terminals. Note that the two interactions constitute a positive feedback.

[18]If one puts the information in this section and that on prostaglandins in note 15 together, it is apparent that a potential positive feedback mechanism exists between prostaglandins and the renin-angiotensin system: ↑ renin release → ↑ [renin] → ↑ [angiotensin II] → ↑ PG release → ↑ [PG] → ↑ renin release → etc. Whether such a positive feedback mechanism does, in fact, ever occur is unclear.

[19]Secretion of the vasodilator prostaglandins is also stimulated by several of the intrarenal vasoconstrictor paracrine agents such as endothelin (see next section in the text); accordingly, the prostaglandins may serve to dampen the effects of these vasoconstrictors as well.

RENAL CLEARANCE

Objectives

The student understands the principles and applications of clearance technique:

1 Defines the term *clearance*
2 States the criteria that must be met for a substance in order for its clearance to be used as a measure of GFR; states which substances are used to measure GFR and ERPF
3 Lists the data required for clearance calculation
4 Given data, calculates C_{In}, C_{PAH}, C_{urea}, $C_{glucose}$, C_{Na}
5 Predicts whether a substance undergoes net reabsorption or net secretion by comparison of its clearance to that of inulin, or by comparison of its rate of filtration to its rate of excretion
6 Given data, calculates net rate of reabsorption or secretion for any substance
7 Given data, calculates fractional excretion of any substance
8 Knows how to estimate GFR from C_{urea} and describes the limitations
9 Describes the limitation of C_{Cr} as a measure of GFR
10 Constructs the curve relating steady-state P_{Cr} to C_{Cr} or P_{urea} to C_{urea}; predicts the changes in P_{Cr} and P_{urea} given a known change in GFR; knows the limitations of this analysis, particularly with regard to urea

The technique known as *clearance* is extremely useful for evaluating renal function both in the laboratory and clinically. The concept of clearance can be difficult to grasp, and so before defining it and developing it in a more formal manner, we shall look at an example of how it is used—the measurement of glomerular filtration rate.

MEASUREMENT OF GFR

Assume there is a substance (let us call it W) that is freely filterable at the renal corpuscle but is not secreted, reabsorbed, or metabolized by the tubules. Then:

$$\frac{\text{Mass of } W \text{ excreted}}{\text{time}} = \frac{\text{Mass of } W \text{ filtered}}{\text{time}} \qquad (3\text{-}1)$$

Since the mass of any solute equals the product of solute concentration and solvent volume,

$$\frac{\text{Mass of } W \text{ excreted}}{\text{time}} = U_W V \qquad (3\text{-}2)$$

where U_W = urine concentration of W
V = urine volume per unit time

Similarly, the mass of W filtered equals the product of the concentration of W in the filtrate and the volume of fluid filtered into Bowman's capsule. Since W is freely filterable, the filtrate concentration of W is the same as the arterial plasma concentration P_W. The volume of plasma filtered per unit time is, by definition, the glomerular filtration rate (GFR). Therefore,

$$\frac{\text{Mass of } W \text{ filtered}}{\text{time}} = P_W \times \text{GFR} \qquad (3\text{-}3)$$

Substituting Eqs. 3-2 and 3-3 into Eq. 3-1:

$$U_W V = P_W \times \text{GFR} \qquad (3\text{-}4)$$

Three of the variables—U_W, V, and P_W—can be measured, and we can solve for GFR:

$$\text{GFR} = \frac{U_W V}{P_W} \qquad (3\text{-}5)$$

The validity of the above analysis depends upon the following characteristics of W:

1. Freely filterable at the renal corpuscle
2. Not reabsorbed
3. Not secreted
4. Not synthesized by the tubules
5. Not broken down by the tubules

A polysaccharide called **inulin** (not insulin) completely fits this description and can be used for the determination of GFR. Consider the following hypothetical situation (Fig. 3-1): To determine your patient's GFR, you infuse inulin at a rate sufficient to maintain plasma concentration constant at 4 mg/L. Urine collected over a 1-h period has a volume of 0.1 L and an inulin concentration of 300 mg/L. What is the patient's GFR?

$$GFR = \frac{U_{In}V}{P_{In}}$$

$$GFR = \frac{300mg/L \times 0.1 \ L/h}{4mg/L}$$

$$GFR = 7.5L/h$$

If any of the five criteria listed above were not valid for inulin, its use would not provide an accurate measure of GFR. For example, if inulin were secreted, which of the following statements would be true?

Calculated GFR would be higher than the true GFR.
Calculated GFR would be lower than the true GFR.

The first statement is correct because the mass of inulin excreted (the numerator in the GFR equation) would represent both filtered *and secreted inulin* and, therefore, would be greater than the filtered inulin.

Unfortunately, measuring GFR with inulin is inconvenient because inulin is not a normally occurring bodily substance and must be administered intravenously at a continuous and constant rate for several hours. Therefore, in

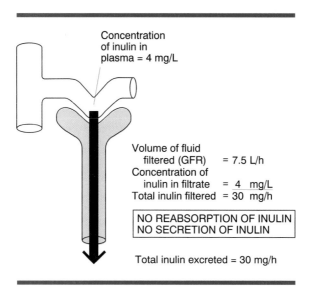

Fig. 3-1 Renal handling of inulin, a substance that is filterable but is neither reabsorbed nor secreted. Therefore, the mass of inulin excreted per unit time is equal to the mass filtered during the same time period. Therefore, as explained in the text, the clearance of inulin is equal to the glomerular filtration rate.

clinical situations the endogenous substance **creatinine** is frequently used to *estimate* GFR. Creatinine is formed from muscle creatine and released into the blood at a fairly constant rate. Consequently, its blood concentration changes little during a 24-h period, so that one need obtain only a single blood sample and a 24-h urine collection.

$$\text{Estimated GFR} = \frac{U_{Cr}V}{P_{Cr}}$$

This is only an estimated GFR because, in humans, creatinine does not meet all five criteria since it is secreted by the tubules. It therefore overestimates the true GFR. However, because the amount secreted is relatively small, the discrepancy is not very large (about 10 percent in normal persons).[1] In a later section we will describe how measurement of plasma creatinine alone without any urine determinations can also be used to estimate GFR more crudely. Use of urea for the same purpose will also be described.

DEFINITION OF CLEARANCE

When we described how inulin could be used to measure GFR (and creatinine to estimate it), we were actually describing the technique known as clearance. First, let us define the term. The **clearance** of a substance is the *volume of plasma* from which that substance is *completely cleared* by the kidneys *per unit time*. Every substance in the plasma has its own distinct clearance value, but the units are always in volume of plasma per time.

Let us apply this to inulin. A certain volume of plasma loses its inulin completely while flowing through the kidney; i.e., a certain volume of plasma is "cleared" of inulin. For inulin, this volume is equal to the GFR since none of the inulin contained in the glomerular filtrate returns to the blood (inulin is not reabsorbed) and none of the plasma that escapes filtration loses any of its inulin (inulin is not secreted). Therefore, a volume of plasma equal to the GFR has been completely cleared of inulin. This volume is called the inulin clearance and is expressed as C_{In}. Accordingly,

$$C_{In} = \text{GFR}$$

What is the glucose clearance? Glucose, like inulin, is freely filtered at the renal corpuscle, so that all the glucose contained in the glomerular filtrate is lost *initially* from the plasma to the tubules. But, unlike inulin, all this filtered glucose is then normally reabsorbed; i.e., it is all returned to the plasma. The net result is that *no* plasma ends up losing glucose; the clearance of glucose is *zero*.

Let us take another example—inorganic phosphate (for the purposes of this example, we will assume that plasma phosphate, P_{PO_4}, is completely filterable). Here are some normal data:

$$GFR = 180 \text{ L/day}$$
$$P_{PO_4} = 1 \text{ mmol/L}$$
$$U_{PO_4}V = 20 \text{ mmol/day}$$

What is the phosphate clearance in this example? The filtered phosphate equals 180 mmol/day (180L/day X 1 mmol/L). Is this the phosphate clearance? The answer is *no*. Clearance does *not* designate a filtered mass. Indeed, it does not designate any mass; it is always a volume per time. The clearance of phosphate is defined as the volume of plasma completely cleared of phosphate per unit time. Is the clearance of phosphate, then, the GFR? Again the answer is no. Certainly, the filtered phosphate contained in the GFR is *initially* lost from the plasma, but much of it—in this example, 160 mmol/day—is reabsorbed, leaving only 20 mmol/day to be excreted in the urine. Is this the phosphate clearance?

Once again the answer is *no*. Clearance is defined not as mass excreted but rather as the volume of plasma supplying that mass per unit time. In other words, the phosphate clearance is the volume of plasma that supplies the excreted 20 mmol; it is this volume that is completely cleared of its phosphate. How much plasma has to be completely cleared of phosphate to supply the 20 mmol? We know from the data that the plasma phosphate concentration equals 1 mmol/L. Therefore, it would take

$$\frac{20 \text{ mmol/day}}{1 \text{ mmol/L}} = 20 \text{ L/day}$$

to supply the excreted phosphate. Clearance of a substance answers the question: How much plasma must be completely cleared to supply the excreted mass of that substance? Accordingly, $C_{PO_4} = 20$ L/day.

BASIC CLEARANCE FORMULA

It should be evident, therefore, that the basic clearance formula for any substance X is

$$C_X = \frac{\text{mass of } X \text{ excreted/time}}{P_X}$$
$$C_X = \frac{U_X V}{P_X}$$

where C_X = clearance of substance X
$\qquad U_X$ = urine concentration of X
$\qquad V$ = urine volume per time
$\qquad P_X$ = arterial plasma concentration of X

C_{In} is a measure of GFR simply because the volume of plasma completely cleared of inulin, i.e., the volume from which the excreted inulin comes, is equal to the volume of plasma filtered. C_{PO_4} must be less than C_{In} because much of the filtered phosphate is reabsorbed; therefore, less plasma was cleared of phosphate than of inulin.

Thus, the following generalization emerges: Whenever the clearance of a freely filterable substance is less than the inulin clearance, tubular reabsorption of that substance must have occurred. This is simply another way of stating that whenever the mass of a substance excreted in the urine is less than the mass filtered during the same period of time, tubular reabsorption must have occurred.

The phrase "freely filterable" is essential in the above generalization. Protein serves as an excellent example. The clearance of protein in a normal person is virtually zero, obviously lower than the C_{In}. However, this does not prove that protein is reabsorbed. The major reason for the zero clearance is that the protein is not filtered. Accordingly, to compare inulin clearance to the clearance of any completely or partially protein-bound substance (calcium, for example), one must use the filterable plasma concentration of the substance rather than the total plasma concentration in the clearance formula.

Is the clearance of creatinine in humans higher or lower than that of inulin? The answer is *higher*. Like inulin, creatinine is freely filtered and not reabsorbed; therefore, a volume of plasma equal to that of the GFR (i.e., the C_{In}) is completely cleared of creatinine. But in addition a small amount of creatinine is secreted. Therefore, some plasma in addition to that filtered is cleared of its creatinine by means of tubular secretion. The clearance formula is precisely the same as that for any other substance:

$$C_{Cr} = \frac{U_{Cr}V}{P_{Cr}}$$

Another generalization emerges: Whenever the clearance of a substance is greater than the inulin clearance, tubular secretion of that substance must have occurred. Again, this is merely another way of stating that whenever the excreted mass exceeds the filtered mass, secretion must be occurring.

Another substance secreted by the proximal tubules is the organic anion **para-aminohippurate (PAH)**. PAH is also filtered at the glomerulus, and when its plasma concentration is fairly low, virtually all the PAH that escapes filtration is secreted. Since PAH is not reabsorbed, the net effect is that all the plasma supplying the nephrons is completely cleared of PAH. (Look back at Fig. 1-9 and you will see that PAH is handled exactly like hypothetical substance X in this figure.) If PAH were completely cleared from all the plasma flowing through the *entire* kidney, its clearance, therefore, would measure the

total renal plasma flow (**RPF**). However, about 10 to 15 percent of the total renal plasma flow supplies nonfiltering and nonsecreting portions of the kidneys (such as peripelvic fat), and this plasma cannot, therefore, lose its PAH by secretion. Accordingly, the PAH clearance actually measures the so-called **effective renal plasma flow** (**ERPF**) and is approximately 85 to 90 percent of the total renal plasma flow. The clearance formula for PAH is, of course:

$$C_{PAH} = \frac{U_{PAH}V}{P_{PAH}} = ERPF$$

Once we have measured the ERPF,[2] we can calculate easily the **effective renal blood flow** (**ERBF**):

$$ERBF = \frac{ERPF}{1 - V_c}$$

where V_c = the blood hematocrit, i.e., the fraction of blood occupied by erythrocytes.

It should be emphasized that C_{PAH} measures ERPF only when plasma PAH is fairly low. If plasma PAH were increased to a level so high that the maximal ability of the tubules to secrete PAH were exceeded, PAH would not be completely removed from the plasma supplying the nephrons and the use of its clearance as a measure of ERPF would be invalid.

Urea clearance C_{urea} can be determined by the usual formula:

$$C_{urea} = \frac{U_{urea}V}{P_{urea}}$$

Urea, like inulin, is freely filterable, but approximately 50 percent of filtered urea is reabsorbed; therefore, C_{urea} will be approximately 50 percent of C_{In}. If the mass of urea reabsorbed were always *exactly* 50 percent of that filtered, could C_{urea} be used to estimate GFR? The answer is *yes*. One would merely multiply the C_{urea} by 2 to obtain a value equal to the GFR. Unfortunately, as will be described in Chapter 5, urea reabsorption varies between 40 and 60 percent of the filtered urea, so that one cannot merely multiply by 2. Nonetheless, the urea clearance is easy to perform clinically and can be used as at least a crude way to evaluate GFR. The creatinine clearance is certainly a better way of estimating GFR, but recall that it is not completely accurate either because of creatinine secretion.

QUANTITATION OF TUBULAR REABSORPTION AND SECRETION USING CLEARANCE

To reiterate, once a method (determination of C_{In}) is available for measuring GFR, it becomes possible to determine whether the overall nephron manifests net reabsorption or net secretion of any given substance. If the clearance of the substance (using the filterable plasma concentration in the calculation) is less than that of inulin, net reabsorption must be occurring; if the clearance of the substance is greater than that of inulin, net secretion exists.

Why the word *net* in the above statements? As we shall see in Chapter 4, some substances can undergo both reabsorption and secretion. Therefore, the finding that the clearance of a filterable substance is less than that of inulin definitely proves reabsorption but does not disprove secretion; secretion may also be occurring but is masked by a greater rate of reabsorption. Similarly, proof of the presence of overall secretion ($C_X > C_{In}$) does not disprove that reabsorption, too, is present but of lesser magnitude than secretion.

Calculation of the magnitude of the *net* reabsorption or secretion in units of mass per time is given for any substance by the following equation:

$$\text{Mass excreted} = \text{mass filtered} + \text{mass secreted} - \text{mass reabsorbed}$$
$$(U_X V) \qquad (\text{GFR} \times P_X)$$

Rearranging terms:

$$\text{Mass filtered} - \text{mass excreted} = (\text{mass reabsorbed} - \text{mass secreted})$$
$$(\text{GFR} \times P_X) \qquad (U_X V)$$

Note that mass reabsorbed and mass secreted are not *directly measured* variables but are derived as a single net value from the measurements of filtered and excreted masses. A positive value (filtered > excreted) quantifies net reabsorption, and a negative value (filtered < excreted) net secretion.

Another common way of quantitating the degree of net reabsorption or net secretion is as **fractional excretion (FE)**. FE answers this question: What fraction of the filtered mass of a substance does the excreted mass represent?

$$\frac{\text{Mass excreted}}{\text{mass filtered}} = \text{fractional excretion}$$

$$\frac{U_X V}{\text{GFR} \times P_X} = \text{FE}_X$$

Thus, for example, an FE_X of 0.23 means that, overall, the mass of X excreted is 23 percent of the mass of X filtered; therefore 77 percent of the filtered X has undergone net reabsorption. An FE_X of 1.5 means that 50 percent *more X* is excreted than was filtered; i.e., secretion is occurring.[3]

PLASMA CREATININE AND UREA CONCENTRATIONS AS INDICATORS OF GFR CHANGES

As described previously, the creatinine clearance is a close approximation of the GFR and is, therefore, a valuable clinical determination.

$$C_{Cr} = \frac{U_{Cr}V}{P_{Cr}}$$

In practice, however, it is far more common to measure plasma creatinine alone and to use this as an *indicator* of GFR. This approach is justified by the fact that most excreted creatinine gains entry to the tubule by filtration. If we ignore the small amount secreted, there should be an excellent inverse correlation between plasma creatinine and GFR, as shown by the following example.

A normal person's plasma creatinine is 10 mg/L. It remains stable because each day the amount of creatinine produced is excreted. One day the GFR suddenly decreases *persistently* by 50 percent because of a blood clot in the renal artery. On that day the person filters only 50 percent as much creatinine as normal so that creatinine excretion is also reduced by 50 percent. (We are ignoring the small contribution of secreted creatinine.) Therefore, assuming no change in creatinine production, the person goes into positive creatinine balance, and the plasma creatinine rises. But despite the persistent 50 percent GFR reduction, the plasma creatinine does not continue to rise indefinitely; rather, it stabilizes at 20 mg/L, i.e., after it has doubled. At this point the person once again is able to excrete creatinine at the normal rate and so remains stable. The reason is that the 50 percent GFR reduction has been counterbalanced by the doubling of plasma creatinine, and filtered creatinine is again normal.

> Original normal state: Filtered creatinine $= 10$ mg/L $\times 180$ L/day
> $\qquad\qquad\qquad\qquad\qquad\qquad = 1800$ mg/day
> New steady state: $\quad$ Filtered creatinine $= 20$ mg/L $\times 90$ L/day
> $\qquad\qquad\qquad\qquad\qquad\qquad = 1800$ mg/day

This is a very important point: In the new steady state, creatinine *excretion* is normal because of the doubling of plasma creatinine concentration. In other words, creatinine excretion is below normal only transiently until plasma creatinine has increased as much proportionally as the GFR has fallen.

What if the GFR then fell to 30 L/day? Again, creatinine retention would occur until a new steady state had been established, i.e., until the person were again filtering 1800 mg/day. What would the new plasma creatinine be?

$$1800 \text{ mg/day} = P_{Cr} \times 30 \text{ L/day}$$
$$P_{Cr} = 60 \text{ mg/L}$$

It should now be clear why a single plasma creatinine measurement is a reasonable indicator of GFR (Fig. 3-2). It is not completely accurate, however, for three reasons: (1) Some creatinine is secreted. (2) There is no way of knowing exactly what the person's original creatinine was when GFR was normal. (3) Creatinine production may not remain completely unchanged.

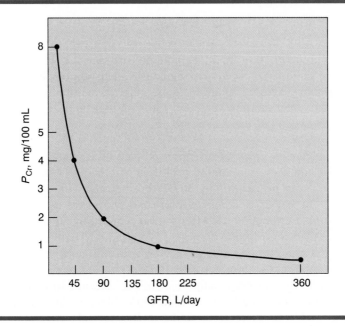

Fig. 3-2   Steady-state relationship between GFR and plasma creatinine, assuming no creatinine is secreted.

Since urea is also handled by filtration, the same type of analysis would indicate that the measurement of plasma urea concentration could serve as an indicator of GFR. However, it is a much less accurate indicator than plasma creatinine because the range of normal plasma urea concentration varies widely, depending on protein intake and changes in tissue catabolism, and because urea is reabsorbed to a *variable* degree. (The fact that it is reabsorbed would not interfere with its use as an indicator if the reabsorption were always a *fixed* percentage of the filtered mass.)

Study questions: 17 to 25

NOTES

[1]Unfortunately, the discrepancy does become large when GFR is very low because secreted creatinine then becomes a significant fraction of excreted creatinine.

[2]To reiterate: C_{PAH} measures ERPF, not RPF, because some PAH escapes filtration and secretion. However, we can measure the amount that has escaped by measuring the concentration of PAH in the renal venous plasma. We can then calculate RPF by using that value in the following equation:

$$RPF = \frac{U_{PAH}V}{arterial_{PAH} - renal\ venous_{PAH}}$$

This equation is simply an example of the law of conservation of mass: What comes in at the renal artery must go out through the renal vein and urine combined.

[3]Note that when inulin is used to measure GFR, the formula for fractional excretion is simply the ratio of C_X/C_{In}:

$$\frac{U_XV/P_X}{U_{In}V/P_{In}} = FE_X$$

Moreover, since urine volume (V) is common to both clearances, it is not even necessary to measure V to calculate a fractional excretion:

$$\frac{U_X/P_X}{U_{In}/P_{In}} = FE_X$$

An analagous double ratio is the key to evaluating, using micropuncture, not *overall* tubular function but the presence of net reabsorption or net secretion in individual nephron segments. Let us take the handling of the hypothetical substance Q by the proximal tubule as an example. A sample of fluid is collected from the end of the proximal tubule in an experimental animal given inulin, and its concentrations of Q and inulin are measured and compared to those of arterial plasma. The fraction of filtered Q remaining at the end of the proximal tubule is given by the ratio:

$$\frac{Tubular\ fluid_Q/Plasma_Q}{Tubular\ fluid_{In}/Plasma_{In}}$$

Let us assume that the value is found to be approximately 0.6; i.e., about 60 percent of the filtered Q remains at the end of the proximal tubule. This means that 40 percent of the filtered Q has been reabsorbed by the proximal tubule.

To determine what the loop of Henle has done, a sample of fluid is collected from the very early distal convoluted tubule and the "double ratio" for it is compared with that for the end of the proximal; it is found to be 1.1, compared to 0.6 for the late proximal, establishing that Q has been secreted into the loop. Similarly, a late distal convoluted sample can be compared with the early distal one to evaluate the net contribution of the distal convoluted tubule, and so on.

BASIC MECHANISMS OF TUBULAR REABSORPTION AND SECRETION

4

Objectives

The student understands the basic mechanisms of tubular reabsorption and secretion:

1　Defines and states the major characteristics of diffusion, facilitated diffusion, primary active transport, secondary active transport (including cotransport and countertransport), endocytosis, and solvent drag

2　States how the mechanisms listed in objective 1 can be combined to achieve active transcellular reabsorption

3　Defines paracellular reabsorption; states the requirements for it to occur; states the orientation of the transtubular potential difference in the proximal tubule, thick ascending limb of Henle's loop, and the more distal segments

4　Describes qualitatively the forces that determine movement of reabsorbed fluid from interstitium into peritubular capillaries; states why the peritubular-capillary hydraulic pressure is low and the oncotic pressure high; states the role of filtration fraction in determining peritubular-capillary oncotic pressure

5　Defines the concept of T_m (either reabsorptive or secretory); given appropriate data, calculates T_m; defines renal plasma threshold; defines splay; states the significance of a T_m being much higher than the usual filtered mass of the substance

6　States how the mechanisms listed in objective 1 can be combined to achieve either paracellular or active transcellular secretion

7　Describes three processes that can produce bidirectional transport of a substance in a single tubular segment; states the consequences of pump-leak systems

8　Contrasts "tight" and "leaky" epithelia

9　States generalizations concerning the usual "division of labor" among tubular segments

This chapter describes the basic principles of tubular reabsorption and secretion. These principles will then be applied to specific substances in Chapters 5 through 10.

CLASSIFICATION OF TRANSPORT MECHANISMS

The molecular mechanisms involved in reabsorption and secretion are basically the same as those involved in movements of molecules across plasma membranes anywhere in the body. The transport of some substances occurs through diffusion, whereas that of others requires mediation by membrane proteins.

Diffusion

This process arises from random molecular motion and requires an electrochemical gradient for net movement to occur; i.e., net diffusion is always "downhill." Lipid-soluble substances can diffuse across the lipid portions of a cell's plasma membranes, whereas ionic diffusion is restricted pretty much to water-filled channels created by the proteins of the plasma membrane. These channels may be highly specific for certain ions; thus, we speak of "sodium channels" or "potassium channels."

Facilitated Diffusion

This process, like diffusion, can produce net movement of a substance only down its electrochemical gradient (thus, the term *diffusion*). However, unlike simple diffusion, the transport depends on interaction of the substance with specific membrane proteins, called *transporters* (or *carriers*), which "facilitate" its movements. The initial event in facilitated diffusion is the binding of the substance to the transporter, followed by a conformational change in the transporter that causes the translocation of the substance across the membrane. The substance then separates from the transporter. Because of the interaction with membrane proteins, facilitated diffusion manifests specificity, saturability, and competition.

Primary Active Transport

In this process, the transported molecule also interacts with membrane transporters and exhibits specificity, saturability, and competition. In contrast to facilitated diffusion, however, primary active transport produces net "uphill" transport, i.e., net transport against an electrochemical gradient. The energy for this active transport comes *directly* from the splitting of ATP. Indeed, the term *primary* specifically denotes that metabolically produced chemical energy is the direct source of the energy for the process. In such cases, membrane-bound ATPase not only splits the ATP to provide energy but also is a component of the actual carrier mechanism. Presently documented primary active transporters are Na,K-ATPase, H-ATPase, H,K-ATPase, and Ca-ATPase.

Secondary Active Transport
(Cotransport and Countertransport)

In this process, two (or sometimes more) substances interact simultaneously with the same specific membrane transporter, and both are translocated across the membrane. The crucial point is that one of the substances undergoes only net "downhill" transport (a form of facilitated diffusion), whereas the other usually manifests net "uphill" movement against its electrochemical gradient. Yet the latter occurs without input of metabolic energy *directly* into the transport process. Rather, the direct source of energy is the energy liberated by the simultaneous downhill movement of the other transported substance. In other words, as one of the substances (often sodium) moves down its electrochemical gradient, the energy released somehow is able to drive the other substance uphill against its electrochemical gradient. The substance moving uphill is said to undergo **secondary active transport** because the active transport is not directly linked to ATP hydrolysis the way primary active transport is.

The term **cotransport**[1] denotes the situation in which the involved substances are moving in the same direction across the membrane, one downhill and the other usually uphill. In **countertransport** the energy liberated by the downhill movement of one of the substances usually produces uphill movement of the second substance in the *opposite* direction. For example, the downhill movement of sodium *into* the cell might provide the energy for uphill movement of hydrogen ion *out of* the cell.

Endocytosis

This process is characterized by the invagination of a portion of the plasma membrane until it becomes completely pinched off and exists as an isolated intracellular membrane-bound vesicle filled with the extracellular fluid it imbibed during its formation. This process offers an important mechanism for the uptake of macromolecules, which may trigger the entire process by binding to specific membrane receptors. Endocytosis, of course, requires energy, and its source is the splitting of ATP.

Solvent Drag

If a membrane contains pores large enough to permit laminar flow during osmosis, then the moving water (the "solvent") will "drag" with it any dissolved solutes which can also enter the pores. Thus the movement of water, due to a water concentration difference across a membrane, can nonspecifically accelerate the movement of many small solutes in the same direction.

TRANSPORT MECHANISMS IN REABSORPTION

We began this discussion of reabsorption and secretion with the statement that they use the same basic mechanisms for transport across any plasma membranes. But we must now face the added complexity that arises when we deal with an *epithelial layer*, such as the renal tubule (or gastrointestinal epithelium, gallbladder epithelium, etc.), rather than the plasma membrane of a single nonepithelial cell (a muscle cell or erythrocyte, for example).

Look at Fig. 4-1 and you will see that there are two potential routes for reabsorptive movement from lumen to interstitium. The first is by movement *between* cells, i.e., across the tight junctions connecting cells, and is called **paracellular**. Paracellular reabsorption can be by diffusion or solvent drag. Diffusion requires that an electrochemical gradient exist for the substance in the reabsorptive direction and that the tight junctions be permeable to the substance. Solvent drag requires the flow of water through relatively "leaky" tight junctions (see below). I shall describe in later chapters how *concentration gradients* for individual substances are created across various tubular segments and also how water flow is induced. I give here a very brief overview of the *electrical potential differences* that exist *between tubular lumen and interstitial fluid* in the various tubular segments.

First, it is essential to recognize that we are dealing here with *transtubular* (or transepithelial) potentials, not simple membrane potentials. The transtubular potential—between tubular lumen and interstitial fluid—is simply the algebraic sum of the individual luminal-membrane and basolateral-membrane potentials.[2] Both these individual membrane potentials are oriented cell-interior negative, i.e., the cell interior is negative relative to both the lumen of the tubule and the interstitial fluid. But the magnitudes of the two

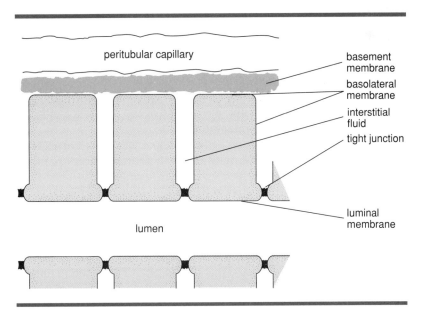

Fig. 4-1 Diagrammatic representation of tubular epithelium. The tight junctions can be visualized three-dimensionally as the sheet of plastic holding together a six-pack of soda, each cell being one of the cans.

plasma-membrane cell-negative potentials may be different, and that is how a transtubular potential—the algebraic sum of the two—is created. In the proximal tubule, the transtubular potential is very small (the reason will be given later in this chapter when we talk about "leaky" epithelia), a few mV lumen-negative relative to the interstitial fluid in the early portions and a few mV lumen-positive in the middle-to-late portions. Because the potential is so low and because it changes along the length of the tubule we will consider the average proximal transtubular potential to be zero; this will allow us to focus mainly on the *concentration* gradients across this tubular segment in considering paracellular diffusion of ions. In the thick ascending limb of Henle's loop the transtubular potential is always significantly lumen-positive and therefore is a force for the paracellular reabsorption of cations—sodium, potassium, calcium, etc. The transtubular potential in most of the more distal segments is significantly lumen-negative and is therefore a force for paracellular reabsorption of anions, chloride being the only one of importance.

The second route for reabsorption is **transcellular** ("across" the cell), in which the reabsorbed substance must cross *two* plasma membranes in its journey from tubular lumen to interstitial fluid—the **luminal** (or apical) **membrane**—separating the luminal fluid from the cell cytoplasm—and the **basolateral** (or contraluminal) **membrane**—separating the cytoplasm from the interstitial fluid. (The substance must, of course, also traverse the cell cytosol between the two membranes.)

Substances that are quite lipid-soluble can traverse both membranes (and the cytosol) by diffusion, and net passive reabsorption occurs by this route, simultaneously with the paracellular route, when a favorable transtubular electrochemical gradient exists for the substance. In contrast, transcellular movement for substances that are poorly lipid-soluble is active. The crucial generalization is as follows: Active net transcellular reabsorption of a substance requires (1) that the luminal and basolateral membranes be asymmetrical for that substance, that is, contain different channels and/or transporters, and (2) that energy be used for the movement of the substance either from lumen into cell or from cell into interstitial fluid.

Let us take sodium reabsorption in the principal cells of the cortical collecting ducts as an example. The first question is whether significant paracellular reabsorption occurs for sodium in this tubular segment. The answer is *no*. Rather, sodium reabsorption is active and transcellular, as illustrated in Fig. 4-2. There is net diffusion of sodium down its electrochemical gradient (see below) from the lumen across the luminal membrane into the cytoplasm through sodium channels. The sodium is then actively transported against its electrochemical gradient across the basolateral membrane into the interstitial fluid. This latter step is a primary active process that uses Na,K-ATPase, found only in the basolateral membrane. Thus, the net unidirectional reabsorption of sodium in this tubular segment occurs because (1) there is asymmetry of the luminal and basolateral membranes—sodium channels in the former and Na,K-ATPase pumps in the latter, and (2) energy is supplied for the basolateral-membrane step by the splitting of ATP by the membrane Na,K-ATPase.

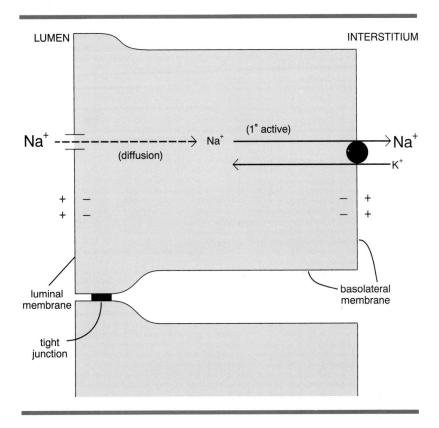

Fig. 4-2 Reabsorption of sodium by the principal cells of the cortical collecting duct. Diffusion into the cell through the sodium channels in the luminal membrane is driven by the sodium concentration gradient (cytosolic sodium concentration being much lower than luminal sodium concentration) and the electrical potential difference (cytosol negative relative to lumen), both ultimately the result of the basolateral primary active Na,K-ATPase "pumps." (These pumps are identical to those in plasma membranes of almost all bodily cells and pump 3 sodiums out of the cell for every 2 potassiums in.) In this tubular segment, the potassium ions actively transported into the cell by the pumps diffuse out through channels in both the luminal and basolateral membranes (see Chapter 8); these paths are not shown in the figure in order to focus only on the fate of sodium.

What may not be apparent from this description is the fact that the luminal event actually depends on the basolateral event. This becomes evident as soon as one recognizes that the net diffusion of sodium across the luminal membrane depends on the existence of a favorable electrochemical gradient—cytoplasmic [Na] < luminal [Na] and/or electric potential difference oriented so that the cell interior is negative relative to the lumen. The crucial point is that the basolateral Na,K-ATPase pump creates this electrochemical gradient across the luminal membrane by keeping the cytoplasmic [Na] low and the cell

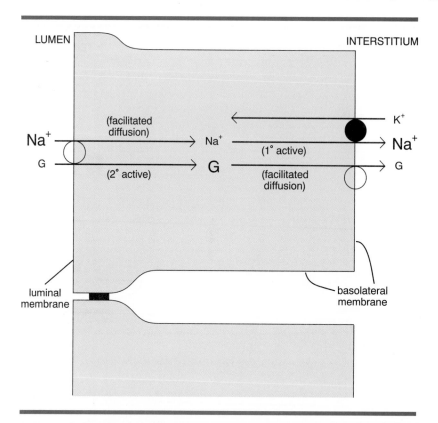

Fig. 4-3 Secondary active reabsorption of glucose by the proximal tubule. Follow this figure by beginning with the primary active Na,K-ATPase pump in the basolateral membrane. You can see how the low intracellular sodium concentration permits the net "downhill" entry of sodium across the luminal membrane, which in turn provides the energy for simultaneous "uphill" glucose movement across this membrane by cotransport with sodium. This figure and Fig. 4-2 together introduce several conventions to be followed in all such transport models: A filled circle denotes a primary active ATPase pump; open circles denote cotransporters and countertransporters; dashed lines denote diffusion through channels. Again, in this figure as in the next, we have ignored the fate of the potassium ions pumped into the cell; it will be described in Chapter 6 when we deal with the proximal tubule.

interior negatively charged, just as plasma-membrane Na,K-ATPase pumps do in virtually all cells of the body.

This example also illustrates how important it is to distinguish between the *transtubular potential*, which drives paracellular diffusion across the epithelium, and the individual luminal- and basolateral-membrane potentials, which influence movements across the individual membranes. The *transtubular potential* in the cortical collecting duct is *lumen-negative* relative to the interstitial fluid, but the *luminal-membrane potential* is *lumen-positive* relative to the cell interior.

Let us take another example, the reabsorption of glucose (Fig. 4-3), which occurs in the proximal tubule. Glucose moves "uphill" from the lumen across the luminal membrane into the cytoplasm by cotransport with sodium. This transporter-mediated movement of glucose is secondary active transport since the energy utilized to drive the uphill movement of glucose across the luminal membrane is derived from the simultaneous downhill movement of sodium along its electrochemical gradient via the cotransporter. So efficient is this cotransporter that the lumen can be virtually cleared of glucose. After entry into the cell, the glucose then exits across the basolateral membrane by sodium-independent facilitated diffusion, this downhill movement being driven by the high-glucose concentration achieved in the cell by the action of the luminal cotransport process. Again we see our crucial requirements for net active transcellular reabsorption being met: (1) The two membranes are asymmetrical with regard to glucose transporters; and (2) energy is added at one membrane, in this case the luminal membrane.

A critical point, easy to miss, is that the entire overall process of glucose reabsorption depends ultimately on the primary active Na,K-ATPase pump in the basolateral membrane. As pointed out earlier, this pump creates the electrochemical gradient required for net downhill movement of sodium across the luminal membrane, and it is this downhill process that provides the energy for the simultaneous uphill movement of the glucose. Now the reader should be able to understand why glucose reabsorption is termed secondary active transport—it is itself uphill ("active") but is "secondary" to (dependent on) "primary" active transport of sodium by the basolateral membrane. Instead of glucose, we could have used amino acids, inorganic phosphate or sulfate, or a variety of organic nutrients as our example, for they, too, undergo secondary active reabsorption by being cotransported with sodium across the luminal membrane in precisely the same manner (see Chapter 5).

One more note about terminology: When referring to transcellular transport, the term *active* is a shorthand way of stating that at least one of the two membrane crossings is achieved by a primary or secondary active process, i.e., that uphill transport against the substance's electrochemical gradient has occurred somewhere between lumen and interstitial fluid. Thus, we say that glucose undergoes active reabsorption.

Fluid Uptake by Peritubular Capillaries

It is worth reemphasizing that this section has dealt so far only with the movement of substances *from tubular lumen to interstitium*, and this generally will be true in the rest of the book as well. There is, of course, one more step required to complete the reabsorption of these solutes and the water that accompanies them: *movement from interstitium into peritubular capillaries*. Here we are dealing once again with the same type of dynamics that occur across all capillaries in the body. Net diffusion is one mechanism for entry into the peritubular capillaries,[3] but the major one is bulk-flow of interstitial fluid, caused by the net balance of hydraulic and oncotic pressures acting across the peritubular capillaries.

Net filtration pressure for fluid movement from interstitium into peritubular capillaries is given by the following equation:

$$P_{net} = P_{Int} + \Pi_{PC} - P_{PC} - \Pi_{Int}$$

where P = hydraulic pressure, Π = oncotic pressure, and the subscripts *Int* and *PC* stand for *interstitium* and *peritubular capillary*. This is the second time we have dealt with capillary dynamics in the kidney, the first being the discussion of glomerular filtration in Chapter 2. The concepts are identical, but of course the locations are different. Glomerular dynamics involve the balance of forces between the glomerular capillaries and Bowman's capsule, whereas the peritubular forces are between the interstitium and the peritubular capillaries. Representative numbers are given for these forces in Table 4-1; the exact numbers are not important or worth memorizing (indeed, precise values are not available for the human kidney) but are given only to illustrate the following basic principles.

The net filtration pressure across the peritubular capillaries always favors net movement *into* the capillaries. There are two major reasons for this fact, both of which were given in Chapter 2: (1) The peritubular-capillary hydraulic pressure is generally quite low (about 20 mmHg) because the blood entering the peritubular capillaries has already had to flow through the afferent arterioles, glomeruli, and efferent arterioles. (2) The oncotic pressure of the plasma entering the peritubular capillaries is higher than that of arterial plasma because the plasma proteins are concentrated by loss of protein-free filtrate during passage through the glomerular capillaries. Early peritubular-capillary oncotic pressure is, therefore, identical to the oncotic pressure at the end of the glomerular capillaries. How much this oncotic pressure exceeds

Table 4-1   Estimated Forces Involved in Movement of Fluid from Interstitium into Peritubular Capillaries*

Forces	mmHg
1 Favoring uptake	
a Interstitial hydraulic pressure, P_{Int}	3
b Oncotic pressure in peritubular capillaries, Π_{PC}	33
2 Opposing uptake	
a Hydraulic pressure in peritubular capillaries, P_{PC}	20
b Interstitial oncotic pressure, Π_{Int}	6
3 Net pressure for uptake (1 − 2)	10

*The values for peritubular-capillary hydraulic and oncotic pressures are for the early portions of the capillary. The oncotic pressure, of course, decreases as protein-free fluid enters it, i.e., as absorption occurs, but would not go below 25 mmHg (the value of arterial plasma) even if all fluid originally filtered at the glomerulus were absorbed.

that of arterial plasma is determined by the filtration fraction—the greater the filtration fraction the more concentrated the protein and the higher the oncotic pressure.

Transport Maximum

Many of the active reabsorptive systems in the renal tubule have a limit, called a **transport maximum** (T_m), to the amounts of material they can transport per unit time, because the membrane proteins responsible for the transport become saturated. An important example is the secondary active transport process for glucose in the proximal tubule. Normal persons do not excrete glucose in their urine because all filtered glucose is reabsorbed, but it is possible to produce urinary excretion of glucose in a completely normal person merely by administering large quantities of glucose directly into a vein (Table 4-2).

Note in Table 4-2 that even after the plasma glucose concentration, and hence the filtered quantity of glucose, has doubled, the urine is still glucose-free, indicating that the T_m for reabsorbing glucose has not yet been reached. But as the plasma glucose and the filtered load continue to rise, glucose finally appears in the urine because all the filtered glucose cannot be reabsorbed. Once the T_m for glucose, which equals 375 mg/min in this person, has been exceeded, any further increase in plasma glucose is accompanied by an equal increase in excreted glucose. The tubules are now reabsorbing all the glucose they can, and any amount filtered in excess of this quantity cannot be reabsorbed and appears in the urine. This is what occurs in patients with diabetes mellitus: Because of an insulin deficiency, the person's plasma glucose may rise to extremely high values; the filtered load of glucose becomes great enough to exceed the T_m, and glucose appears in the urine. There is nothing wrong in this situation with the tubular transport mechanism for glucose; it is simply unable to reabsorb the huge filtered load.

Table 4-2 Experimental Data Obtained for Calculation of Glucose T_m*

Time, min	GFR, ml/min	P_G, mg/ml	Filtered glucose (GFR × P_G), mg/min	Excreted glucose (U_GV), mg/min	Reabsorbed glucose (filtered − excreted), mg/min
0 Begin glucose infusion	125	1.0	125	0	125
26–40	125	2.0	250	0	250
100–110	125	4.0	500	125	375
130–140	125	5.0	625	250	375

*GFR = glomerular filtration rate; P_G = plasma glucose concentration; U_G = urine glucose concentration; V = urine volume per time.

To add one more level of complexity, let us return to the experiment in which glucose was infused. Additional data were obtained for minutes 60 to 100 but were not shown in Table 4-2. They are as follows:

Time, min	GFR, ml/min	P_G mg/ml	Filtered glucose, mg/min	Excreted glucose, mg/min	Reabsorbed glucose, mg/min
60–80	125	2.8	350	20	330
80–100	125	3.5	436	76	360

Now we see that glucose began to be excreted in the urine *before* the true T_m of 375 mg/min was reached. The plasma concentration at which glucose first appears in the urine is known as the **renal plasma threshold** for glucose. The appearance of glucose in the urine before the T_m is reached is called **splay**. A major explanation of splay is as follows: Not all nephrons have the same T_m for glucose, so that some may be spilling glucose at a time when others have not yet reached their individual T_ms.

Except for our experimental subject who received intravenous glucose, the plasma glucose in normal persons never becomes high enough to cause urinary excretion of glucose, because the T_m for glucose is much greater than necessary for normal filtered loads. This relationship between T_m and filtered amount is also true for many other organic nutrients. Therefore, the filtered amounts of all these substances are normally *completely* reabsorbed, none appearing in the urine. For these substances, like substance Z in our earlier example (Fig. 1-9), it is as though the kidneys did not exist because they do not normally eliminate them from the body at all. Therefore, the kidneys do not help *regulate* the plasma concentrations of these substances. Rather, the kidneys merely maintain whatever plasma concentrations already exist, generally the result of hormonal regulation of nutrient metabolism. In contrast, the reabsorption rates for water and many ions, although also very high, are regulatable and so the kidneys can alter the amounts reabsorbed and hence excreted.

TRANSPORT MECHANISMS IN TUBULAR SECRETION

Tubular secretory processes transport substances across the tubular epithelium into the lumen, i.e., in the direction opposite to tubular reabsorption, and constitute a second pathway into the tubule, the first pathway being glomerular filtration. The term tubular secretion denotes only the *direction* of transport; the specific membrane-transport mechanisms by which tubular secretion is achieved are precisely the same as those described in the first section of this chapter.

The overall secretory process for any given substance begins with its diffusion out of the peritubular capillaries into the interstitial fluid, from which it makes its way into the lumen by crossing either the tight junctions—the paracellular route—or, in turn, the basolateral and luminal membranes of the cell—the transcellular route.

Passive secretion—either paracellular or transcellular—can occur by diffusion when there is a favoring electrochemical gradient for the substance between the interstitial fluid and tubular lumen and the plasma membranes and/or tight junctions are permeable to the substance.

In the case of active secretion, which is always transcellular, the requirements are precisely the same as for active reabsorption, only the direction is reversed: (1) differences in the transport characteristics of the two membranes, and (2) the input of energy at one of them. In most cases (an example is given in Fig. 4-4), the secreted substance is actively transported across the basolateral membrane by a primary or secondary active process, and the resulting high intracellular concentration then drives "downhill" movement across the luminal membrane, either through channels or by facilitated diffusion. In other cases, the active step is at the luminal membrane and the downhill step at the basolateral membrane.

Since the first step in the tubular secretion of a substance is diffusion of the substance from peritubular capillary into interstitial fluid, you might suppose that substances mainly bound to plasma proteins could not undergo tubular secretion. However, such is not the case. There are always some free molecules of the substance in equilibrium with those bound to plasma proteins, and as the free molecules diffuse out of the capillary, others come off the plasma proteins, by mass action, to take their place. This happens rapidly enough so that in those cases in which an active secretory system exists for a protein-bound substance, almost all the substance originally bound to the protein can undergo secretion, often during a single passage of blood through the kidneys.

Among the most important secretory processes are those for potassium and hydrogen ions, and these will be discussed in Chapters 8 and 9, respectively. (As an appetizer, go back to Fig. 4-2 and simply insert a potassium channel in the luminal membrane so that some of the potassium entering across the basolateral membrane via the Na,K-ATPase pumps can diffuse across the luminal membrane; voilà, this cell now not only actively reabsorbs sodium but also actively secretes potassium.)

In the proximal tubule, there are also several active secretory systems for organic anions and cations (Chapter 5).

BIDIRECTIONAL TRANSPORT

In the preceding sections, the adjective *net* was frequently used in reference to tubular reabsorption or secretion and was always implicit even when absent. The fact is that only rarely, if ever, does any transported substance manifest purely unidirectional flux across the tubule totally unopposed by a flux in the other direction.

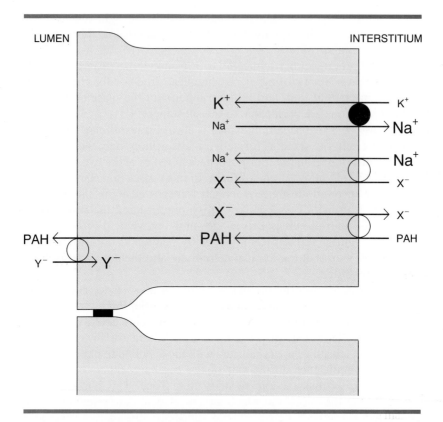

Fig. 4-4 An example of an actively secreted substance—the organic anion *p*-amino-hippurate (PAH). This occurs in the proximal tubule. For the moment start at the bottom right of the figure. PAH, which has diffused out of the peritubular capillaries, undergoes secondary active transport into the cell across the basolateral membrane via counter-transport with another organic anion, X^- (usually α-ketoglutarate). The energy for this step is supplied by X^- moving "downhill" from cell to interstitial fluid. The luminal exit step for PAH is "downhill" and is by countertransport with any of a large number of organic anions (denoted by Y^-). Now back up and you'll see that the entire process is indirectly dependent on the basolateral-membrane Na,K-ATPase pumps: (1) These pumps, as always, create a Na^+ concentration gradient across the basolateral mem-brane; (2) this gradient drives the "downhill" movement of sodium into the cell by a cotransporter that utilizes the energy from the process simultaneously to move X^- "uphill" into the cell. i.e., X^- undergoes secondary active transport; (3) as described above, the X^- moving back "downhill" across the basolateral membrane then supplies the energy to transport PAH actively into the cell. Thus, X^- is simply being recycled across the basolateral membrane. It should also be clear why the PAH transport is an example of what is termed "tertiary" active transport. PAH secretion is typical of a large number of organic anions, as discussed in Chapter 5, although the details may differ from substance to substance.

One important reason for bidirectional transport is apparent from reconsideration of the example in Fig. 4-4. Note that the overall active secretory process achieves a concentration of PAH higher in the lumen than in the interstitial fluid. This difference, of course, favors a net movement of PAH in the *reabsorptive* direction by paracellular diffusion, so that if the tight junctions are at all permeable to PAH such movement will occur. In an analogous manner, active reabsorptive processes tend to establish a concentration lower in the lumen than in the interstitial fluid, and this concentration difference favors passive paracellular secretion.[4]

Thus we are dealing with so-called **pump-leak systems**, in which the active-transport system (the "pump") creates a diffusion gradient that opposes its own action by favoring back-diffusion. Since this back-diffusion occurs solely as an indirect result of the pump's activity and since the *net* flux will, therefore, always be in the direction of the pump, we do not usually dignify the back-diffusion with the terms *reabsorption* or *secretion*. In other words, in reference to Fig. 4-4, we say simply that PAH is handled by secretion and we do not call any passive back-flux reabsorption. To take the sodium pattern of Fig. 4-2 as another example, we say simply that sodium is reabsorbed, and we do not assign the term *secretion* to any passive back-flux into the lumen.

The "leak" component of epithelial pump-leak systems is, however, a very important determinant of the maximal concentration gradients that can be established across the epithelial layer. Thus, to refer again to Fig. 4-2, the more permeable the epithelium is to sodium, the more difficult it will be for the active reabsorptive mechanism to decrease luminal sodium concentration below interstitial-fluid sodium concentration. Analogously, an active secretory mechanism is less able to raise the luminal concentration of the transported substance above its interstitial-fluid concentration when the permeability of the epithelial layer to that substance is very high.

For most mineral ions and many organic molecules, the major route for the "leak" in pump-leak systems is paracellular. On the basis of the relative permeabilities of the tight junctions, as manifested by their electrical resistances, various epithelia are classified as "leaky" or "tight." Leaky epithelia include the proximal tubules (as well as the epithelia of the small intestine and gallbladder). Tight epithelia include the distal convoluted tubules and collecting ducts.

To reiterate, leaky epithelia do not achieve large ionic concentration gradients between lumen and interstitial fluid. In addition, only relatively low electrical potentials exist across them (because the passive leaks "short-circuit" the potentials), and they also have high water permeabilities. In contrast, tight epithelia can exhibit very large concentration differences between tubular lumen and interstitium, large transcellular potential differences, and low water permeabilities. These characteristics should be kept in mind when we discuss, in subsequent chapters, the transport of ions and water by the proximal (leaky) and more distal (tight) segments of the tubule.

Pump-leak systems are not the only cause of bidirectional transport within a single tubular segment. Another reason is that a tubular segment may contain opposing pathways, often residing in distinct cell types in the segment. (For example, in the cortical collecting duct one cell type reabsorbs bicarbonate and a second type secretes it.) Alternatively, a single cell type may contain "reversible" transporters for a substance. In both cases the tubular segment may therefore manifest net secretion or net reabsorption, depending on the physiological circumstances.

Finally, for many substances, a particular tubular segment may always carry out only net reabsorption or only net secretion, but other tubular segments may do just the opposite. For example, a substance may be secreted into the proximal tubule but reabsorbed from the collecting duct. In such cases, the relative magnitudes of the opposing processes in the different tubular segments determine whether the overall effect of the entire tubule is reabsorption or secretion.

REGULATION OF MEMBRANE CHANNELS AND TRANSPORTERS

I emphasized earlier in this chapter that tubular reabsorption and/or secretion of many substances is under physiological control. For most of these substances the control is achieved by regulation of the membrane proteins involved in transport—channels and transporters—by hormones, neurotransmitters, and paracrine/autocrine agents. In addition, channels can also respond to changes in local membrane potential, mechanical force, and intracellular ion concentrations. The responses of the channels and transporters (and hence of the cell) to these regulatory messengers are the result of the variety of possible events summarized in Table 4-3.

A very large number of renal studies are directed toward identification of the specific channels and transporters in individual tubular segments and elucidation of the molecular mechanisms by which these proteins function and are regulated. Comprehensive coverage of these mechanisms is, of course, well beyond the scope of this book.

Table 4-3 Summary of Ways by Which Regulatory Messengers Alter the Activity or Number of the Proteins that Function as Plasma-Membrane Channels and Transporters*

1	Binding of regulatory ligands to the protein
2	Covalent modification of the protein by phosphorylation or dephosphorylation
3	Translocation of the protein from intracellular stores to the plasma membrane
4	Endocytosis of the protein from the plasma membrane
5	Changes in the rates of synthesis or degradation of the protein

*The signal transduction mechanisms by which the regulatory messengers bring about these responses in renal cells are the same as those employed by other cells in the body—cyclic AMP, cyclic GMP, membrane phospholipids, gene induction, and so on.

TUBULAR DIVISION OF LABOR

As you proceed through subsequent chapters, you should keep in mind several generalizations which deal with the reabsorption and secretion of individual substances by the various tubular segments. As we have seen, in order to excrete waste products adequately the GFR must be very large. This means though, that the filtered loads of all the other low-molecular-weight plasma solutes are also very large. The proximal tubule has the primary role of recovering these filtered loads by marked reabsorption. This segment has been called a "mass reabsorber" since for every reabsorbed substance the proximal tubule does most of the reabsorbing, the range varying from 50 to 100 percent of the filtered loads, depending on the substance. Similarly, with one major exception (potassium), the proximal tubule is the major site of solute secretion.

Henle's loop, particularly the thick ascending limb, also reabsorbs relatively large quantities of the major ions and, to a lesser extent, water (15 to 35 percent of the filtered loads). Extensive reabsorption by the proximal tubule and Henle's loop ensures that the masses of solutes and the volume of water entering the more distal segments are relatively small.

The tubular segments beyond Henle's loop then do the fine tuning for most substances, determining the final amounts excreted in the urine by adjusting their rates of reabsorption and, in a few cases, secretion. It should not be surprising, therefore, that most (but not all) homeostatic controls are exerted on the more distal segments.

There are basically two ways to organize the teaching of renal physiology. One is to focus on each individual tubular segment in turn and describe in one place all the things it does; this provides the student with a feel for the integrated functioning of each tubular segment. The other approach, which we will follow, focuses on individual substances, following each along the nephron. In this way you will learn in Chapter 6 what the various tubular segments do to sodium, in Chapter 8 what they do to potassium, and so on. Therefore, in order to achieve the goal of the first approach, as well, Appendix A provides complete summaries of all the reabsorptive and secretory activities performed by the individual tubular segments, as covered in the various chapters. These summaries contain only material presented in the text, and they therefore provide an excellent review when you have completed the book.

Study questions: 26 and 27

NOTES

[1]Several terminologies are used to describe the transporters in these coupled systems. The one employed in this book uses the terms *cotransporter* and *countertransporter*. The other uses *symport* instead of cotransporter, and *antiport* instead of countertransporter. The latter terminology also refers to the transporter that mediates facilitated diffusion not coupled to movement of another substance as a *uniport*.

[2]The precise origins of the renal membrane potentials can be quite complex. Suffice it to say that both ionic diffusion and electrogenic transporters contribute to them. (See Palmer and Sackin in Suggested Readings.)

[3]For example, diffusion is involved for those substances, like glucose, that are reabsobed in greater proportion than water. Their concentration becomes higher in the interstitial fluid than in the peritubular-capillary plasma, and this causes net diffusion into the capillaries.

[4]In the case of ions, the active transport may not only create an opposing concentration gradient but an opposing electrical gradient as well. Thus active reabsorption of sodium tends to make the lumen negative relative to the intersitium, thereby creating an electrical force favoring passive back-leakage into the tubule.

RENAL HANDLING OF ORGANIC SUBSTANCES

5

Objectives

The student understands the renal handling of certain organic substances:

1 States the major characteristics of the proximal-tubular systems for active reabsorption of organic nutrients
2 Describes the renal handling of proteins and small peptides
3 Describes the renal handling of urea
4 Describes the active proximal secretory system for organic anions
5 Describes the renal handling of urate
6 Describes the active proximal secretory system for organic cations
7 Describes, in general terms, the renal handling of weak acids and bases, including the contributions of glomerular filtration, active proximal secretion, and passive movements secondary to water reabsorption or pH changes; given any change in luminal pH, predicts the change in net transtubular movement for a substance with a particular pK

Subsequent chapters of this book will deal almost exclusively with the renal handling of inorganic substances since homeostatic regulation of their excretion constitutes the kidney's major physiological role. However, as pointed out in Chapter 1, another major renal function is the excretion of organic waste products, foreign chemicals, and their metabolites. Moreover, reabsorptive processes must exist to prevent massive excretion of filtered organic nutrients. An analysis of the renal transport pathways for all these organic substances is well beyond the scope of this book, but this chapter briefly describes certain of the major ones.

ACTIVE PROXIMAL REABSORPTION OF ORGANIC NUTRIENTS: GLUCOSE, AMINO ACIDS, ETC.

The proximal tubule is the major site for reabsorption of the large quantities of organic nutrients filtered each day by the renal corpuscles. These include glucose, amino acids, acetate, Krebs cycle intermediates, certain water-soluble vitamins, lactate, acetoacetate, β-hydroxybutyrate, and still others. The characteristics of glucose reabsorption described in examples used in Chapter 4 (see Fig. 4-3) are typical of the transport processes for most of them:

1. They are active in that they can reabsorb their respective solutes against electrochemical gradients. Indeed, the intraluminal concentration of the substance in many cases can be reduced virtually to zero; i.e., reabsorption can be 100 percent complete.[1]
2. The "uphill" step is across the luminal membrane, usually via cotransport with sodium.[2]
3. They manifest T_ms (T_m = transport maximum) that are usually well above the amounts *normally* filtered. Accordingly, the kidneys protect against loss of the substances but do not help set their plasma concentrations. As we saw for glucose in diabetic persons, the plasma concentration of these substances may increase so much under abnormal conditions that the filtered load exceeds the reabsorptive T_m and large quantities become lost in the urine. Good examples are acetoacetate and β-hydroxybutyrate in patients with severe uncontrolled diabetes.
4. They manifest specificity. This statement means that a variety of different membrane transporters exist for them. But there is by no means a one-to-one correspondence since two or more closely related substances may use the same transporter. For example, the amino acid transporters are distinct from those for glucose and other monosaccharides, but there are not 20 separate transporters, one for each amino acid. Rather there is one for arginine, lysine, and ornithine; another for glutamate and aspartate; and so on. Shared pathways allow for competition among those substances utilizing any given pathway.
5. They are inhibitable by a variety of drugs and diseases. There are persons with genetic defects manifested as a deficit in one or more of these proximal reabsorptive systems. In some cases, the deficit may be highly specific (e.g., involving only one amino acid), whereas in others, multiple systems may be involved (e.g., glucose and many amino acids). This range of defects is also seen when the deficit is due to an external agent (lead toxicity, for example) rather than to a genetic abnormality.

PROTEINS AND PEPTIDES

The proximal tubule is also the major site for protein reabsorption, and it is treated separately here to emphasize its importance and the fact that its reabsorptive pathway is quite different from those for the nutrients described in the preceding section. Indeed, as we shall see, the term *reabsorption*, though widely used, is really a misnomer.

As mentioned, there is a very small amount of protein in the glomerular filtrate. The normal concentration approximates 10 mg/L, about 0.02 percent of plasma albumin concentration (50 g/L). Yet because of the huge volume of fluid filtered per day, this concentration is not negligible.

$$\text{Total filtered protein} = \text{GFR} \times \text{filtrate concentration of protein}$$
$$= 180 \text{ L/day} \times 10 \text{ mg/L}$$
$$= 1.8 \text{ g/day}$$

If none of this protein were reabsorbed, the entire 1.8 g would be lost in the urine. In fact, almost all the filtered protein is reabsorbed so that the excretion of protein in the urine is normally only 100 mg/day. The mechanism by which protein is reabsorbed is easily saturated, however, so any large increase in filtered protein resulting from increased glomerular permeability can cause the excretion of large quantities of protein.

The initial step in protein reabsorption is endocytosis at the luminal membrane. This energy-requiring process is triggered by the binding of filtered protein molecules to specific receptors on the luminal membrane. Therefore, the rate of endocytosis is increased in proportion to the concentration of protein in the glomerular filtrate until a maximal rate of vesicle formation, and thus the T_m for protein reabsorption, is reached. The pinched-off intracellular vesicles resulting from endocytosis merge with lysosomes, whose enzymes degrade the protein to low-molecular-weight fragments, mainly individual amino acids. These end products then exit the cells across the basolateral membrane into the interstitial fluid, from which they gain entry to the peritubular capillaries.

It should be evident from this description that the term *reabsorption*, in reference to protein handling, is not really accurate, since the intact protein molecules themselves are not actually moving from lumen to peritubular capillary but are catabolized inside the tubular cells. Nevertheless, the important point is that the filtered proteins are not excreted in the urine and their amino acids are retained in the body.

Discussions of the renal handling of protein logically tend to focus on albumin, since it is by far the most abundant plasma protein. There are, of course, many other plasma proteins, and it should be emphasized here that many of these proteins, being smaller than albumin, are filtered to a greater degree than albumin. For example, growth hormone (m.w. = 20,000) is approximately 60 percent filterable. This means that relatively large fractions of these smaller plasma proteins are filtered and then degraded in tubular cells. Accordingly, the kidneys are major sites of catabolism of many plasma proteins, including polypeptide hormones, and decreased rates of degradation occurring in renal disease may result in elevated plasma hormone concentrations.

Small polypeptides, such as angiotensin II, are handled differently than proteins although the end result is the same—the catabolism of the peptide and preservation of its amino acids. They are completely filterable at the renal corpuscles and are then catabolized mainly into amino acids within the proximal-tubular *lumen* by peptidases located on the luminal plasma membrane. The amino acids (as well as any di- and tripeptides generated by this process) are then reabsorbed.

Finally, it should be noted that in certain types of renal damage, proteins released from tubular cells rather than filtered at the renal corpuscles may appear in the urine and provide important diagnostic information.

UREA

Just as glucose provides an excellent example of an actively reabsorbed solute, urea, the primary end product of protein catabolism, provides an example of passive reabsorption, driven by concentration gradients across the tubule.[3]

Since urea is freely filtered at the renal corpuscle, its concentration in Bowman's capsule is identical to its concentration in peritubular-capillary plasma. Then, as the fluid flows along the proximal convoluted tubule, water reabsorption occurs, increasing the concentration of any intratubular solute, such as urea, not undergoing active reabsorption. As a result, the concentration of urea in the tubular lumen becomes greater than in the peritubular-capillary plasma. This concentration gradient causes the net diffusion of urea from tubular lumen to interstitial fluid and then into peritubular capillaries. Thus, urea reabsorption is completely dependent on water reabsorption, which establishes the concentration gradient. Approximately 50 percent of the filtered urea is reabsorbed by the proximal convoluted tubule.

Virtually all of the unreabsorbed urea remains in the tubule as the fluid flows through Henle's loop, the distal convoluted tubule, the cortical collecting duct, and the first part of the medullary collecting duct, since all these segments are relatively impermeable to urea.[4] The reabsorption of water in these segments causes a progressively marked increase in luminal urea concentration. Then, in the inner medulla, this high luminal urea concentration drives urea reabsorption—via facilitated-diffusion urea transporters in both the apical and basolateral membranes—out of the collecting duct into the medullary interstitial fluid. About another 10 percent of the filtered load of urea is reabsorbed at this site; adding this to the 50 percent reabsorbed proximally gives a total of 60 percent of the filtered load reabsorbed by the overall tubule.

This figure applies in situations where water reabsorption by the tubule is maximal. Significantly less of the filtered urea is reabsorbed when water reabsorption is reduced. There are two reasons for this: (1) The concentration gradient for urea reabsorption is created by water reabsorption, and so when water reabsorption is reduced, a smaller urea gradient is created. (2) The urea facilitated-diffusion transporter in the inner medullary collecting ducts is stimulated by the hormone, antidiuretic hormone, which, as will be discussed in Chapter 6, is also the major stimulator of collecting-duct water reabsorption.

ACTIVE PROXIMAL SECRETION OF ORGANIC ANIONS

The proximal tubule actively secretes a large number of different organic anions, both endogenously produced and foreign (see Table 5-1 for a partial listing). Many of the organic anions handled by this system are also filterable

Table 5-1 Some Organic Anions Actively Secreted by the Proximal Tubule

Endogenous substances	Drugs
Bile salts	Acetazolamide
Fatty acids	Chlorothiazide
Hippurates	Ethacrynate
Hydroxybenzoates	Furosemide
Oxalate	Penicillin
Prostaglandins	Probenecid
Urate	Saccharin
	Salicylates
	Sulfonamides

at the renal corpuscles, and so the amount secreted proximally adds to that which gains entry to the tubule via glomerular filtration. Others, however, are extensively bound to plasma proteins and so undergo glomerular filtration only to a limited extent; accordingly, proximal-tubular secretion constitutes the only significant mechanism for their excretion (recall from Chapter 4 that binding to plasma proteins does not generally impede active tubular secretion).

The active secretory pathway for organic anions in the proximal tubule has a relatively low specificity; i.e., a single kind of transporter (or possibly several closely related ones) is responsible for the secretion of all the organic anions listed in Table 5-1 and many more. The relatively nondiscriminating nature of this sytem accounts for its ability to eliminate from the body so many drugs and other foreign environmental chemicals.[5]

The most intensively studied organic anion secreted by this pathway is **para-aminohippurate (PAH)**, the substance, as we saw in Chapter 3, that is used for the measurement of effective renal plasma flow. PAH served as our example of tubular secretion in Chapter 4 (Fig. 4-4); it is actively transported into proximal-tubular cells across the basolateral membrane, and the resulting high intracellular concentration then provides the gradient for the facilitated diffusion of PAH across the luminal membrane into the tubular lumen.

As the plasma concentration of an anion secreted by this system increases, so does the rate of secretion (until the T_m for that substance is reached). This provides a mechanism for homeostatically regulating the endogenous organic anions handled by the system and for speeding the excretion of foreign organic anions.

PAH is typical, in yet another way, of many of the organic anions secreted proximally: It undergoes no significant additional transport anywhere along the nephron. In contrast, some of the other organic anions secreted by the proximal tubule can undergo other forms of transport both in the proximal tubule and in more distal segments. The most important of these is *passive* tubular reabsorption or secretion, which will be described in the last section of this chapter.

Urate

An example of the renal handling of organic anions which is particularly important for clinical medicine is urate, of which an elevated plasma concentration can cause gout. The major form of uric acid in plasma is ionized urate. Urate is not protein-bound and so is freely filterable at the renal corpuscles. Urate undergoes active tubular secretion, mainly in the proximal tubule, by the mechanisms just described. In addition, however, it is also actively *reabsorbed*, again mainly in the proximal tubule.[6] The rate of tubular reabsorption is normally much greater than the rate of tubular secretion, and so the mass of urate excreted per unit time is only a small fraction of the mass filtered.

Although urate reabsorption is greater than secretion, the secretory process is the one that is homeostatically controlled to maintain relative constancy of plasma urate. In other words, if plasma urate begins to increase because of increased urate production, the active proximal secretion of urate is stimulated, thereby increasing urate excretion.

Given these mechanisms of renal urate handling, the reader should be able to deduce the three ways by which altered renal function can lead to decreased urate excretion and hence increased plasma urate, as in gout: (1) decreased filtration of urate secondary to decreased GFR; (2) excessive reabsorption of urate; and (3) diminished secretion of urate.

ACTIVE PROXIMAL SECRETION OF ORGANIC CATIONS

Proximal tubules possess an active transport system (or several closely related systems) for organic cations that is analogous to that for organic anions: It is relatively nonspecific in that it transports a large number of foreign and endogenous substances (Table 5-2), which compete with each other for transport, and it manifests a T_m limitation.

The proximal secretion of organic cations, as of organic anions, is particularly critical for the excretion of those substances extensively bound to plasma

Table 5-2 Some Organic Cations Actively Secreted by the Proximal Tubule

Endogenous substances	Drugs
Acetylcholine	Atropine
Choline	Isoproterenol
Creatinine	Cimetidine
Dopamine	Meperidine
Epinephrine	Morphine
Guanidine	Procaine
Histamine	Quinine
Serotonin	Tetraethyl ammonium
Norepinephrine	
Thiamine	

proteins and not filterable at the renal corpuscle. However, again similar to the case for the organic anions, many of the organic cations secreted by the proximal tubules are not protein-bound and therefore also undergo glomerular filtration as well as tubular secretion; creatinine is a good example.

Finally, and again analogous to the story for organic anions, some organic cations are not only actively secreted by the proximal tubules but may also undergo other forms of tubular handling, mainly passive reabsorption or secretion, a subject to which we now turn.

PASSIVE REABSORPTION OR SECRETION OF WEAK ORGANIC ACIDS AND BASES

Many organic anions and cations are the ionized forms, respectively, of weak acids and bases. Quite apart from any active tubular handling—mainly the active proximal secretion described in the previous two sections—such substances, in their nonionized forms, may also undergo *passive reabsorption* or *passive secretion*, depending on several conditions, the most important being the pH of the urine. To be specific, many weak acids undergo passive tubular secretion when the urine is highly alkaline but passive tubular reabsorption when it is acidic. The opposite pattern is seen for many weak organic bases.

To understand what accounts for this pH dependency, one must realize that the renal-tubular epithelium, like other biological membranes, is mainly a lipid barrier. Accordingly, highly lipid-soluble substances can penetrate it fairly readily by diffusion. One of the major determinants of lipid solubility is the polarity of a molecule; the more polar, the less lipid-soluble. Now, a weak acid exists as a polar ion in alkaline solution and as a nonpolar molecule in acid solution:

$$A^- + H^+ \rightleftharpoons AH$$

In contrast, for weak bases, the ionic form is favored in acid solutions.

$$B + H^+ \rightleftharpoons BH^+$$

Accordingly, the diffusible form of weak acids is generated in acidic fluid, whereas the diffusible form of weak bases is generated in alkaline fluid.

Let us now apply these principles to the *passive* renal transport of a weak acid. In this discussion, we will ignore the fact that the substance, in its nonionized form, may also undergo active proximal secretion by the organic anion system.

Let us assume that the substance is not protein-bound and so its concentration in Bowman's capsule is identical to that in peritubular-capillary plasma. Moreover, because the pH of the glomerular filtrate is identical to that of peritubular-capillary plasma, the relative proportions of A^- and AH are also the same in the two fluids. As the filtered fluid flows along the tubule, water is reabsorbed, and this removal of solvent concentrates both A^- and AH, thereby creating lumen-to-plasma concentration gradients favoring net reabsorption by diffusion (exactly as described for urea). However, since only AH can penetrate the membrane to any great extent, only this form is reabsorbed. Simultaneously, and this is really the crucial point, secretion of hydrogen ions into the lumen lowers the luminal pH and favors, by mass action, the generation of AH, which can then diffuse along its concentration gradient from lumen to peritubular plasma (Fig. 5-1, top). In other words, water reabsorption is one factor that helps create the concentration gradient required for passive reabsorption of AH, but luminal acidification, by generating the diffusible form—AH—of the substance from the nondiffusible form—A⁻—is even more important in creating the gradient.

The story is even more interesting, however, for as we shall see in Chapter 9, the tubular fluid can be made *alkaline* rather than more acid under certain circumstances. This would shift the intraluminal reaction toward generation of A⁻ at the expense of AH, and the resulting decrease in luminal AH would, of

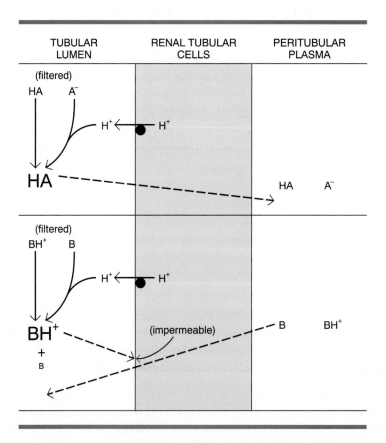

Fig. 5-1 Acidification of the luminal fluid creates, by mass action, the gradients that drive net passive reabsorption (– –) of weak acids (top) and net passive secretion (– –) of weak bases (bottom). The source of the secreted hydrogen ions is discussed in Chapter 9.

course, reduce the gradient for net reabsorption. Indeed, luminal AH might actually fall below peritubular-capillary plasma AH, thereby establishing a gradient for net passive *secretion* rather than reabsorption of AH. Thus, the passive reabsorption of weak organic acids is inversely related to urine pH, and passive secretion may be seen when the urine is alkaline.

We have been dealing with these concepts only qualitatively. The quantitative relationship is determined by the pK of the acid and the pH of the tubular fluid. For example, an acid with a pK well below the lowest tubular-fluid pH achievable—4.4—would always exist within the tubule almost entirely in the anionic (nondiffusible) form and thus always undergo relatively little passive reabsorption. In contrast, an organic acid with a pK of 6 would exhibit a marked increase in the degree of passive reabsorption if intratubular-fluid pH were lowered from 7 to 5, since the nonionized (diffusible) form would go from 10 percent of the total to 90 percent. Importantly, because pH changes are, as we shall see, greatest in the more distal tubular segments, these segments are the major sites for such pH-dependent passive transport.

Let us apply these same concepts to the passive renal-tubular handling of weak bases (Fig. 5-1, bottom): When the tubular fluid is highly acidic, the generation of BH^+ from B is favored. The BH^+ cannot diffuse out of the lumen because of its charge, but the lowering of intraluminal B favors net passive secretion of B from peritubular-capillary plasma into the lumen. Conversely, when the urine is alkaline, generation of B within the lumen is favored, and a gradient is established for net passive reabsorption. Thus, weak bases are passively reabsorbed when the urine is alkaline but may be passively secreted when it is acid.

It must be reemphasized that this section has focussed only on *passive* reabsorption and secretion of these substances. The fact is, as described earlier in this chapter, *active* secretory mechanisms also exist—in the proximal tubule—for the anionic and cationic forms of many weak acids and bases. Accordingly, these forms may be actively secreted into the proximal-tubular lumen followed by either passive reabsorption or passive secretion of the nonionized forms there and, more commonly, in the subsequent tubular segments, depending in part on urine flow rate but mainly on the change in luminal pH occurring along the tubule.

In summary, the excretion of a weak acid or base reflects the following factors:

1. The amount filtered at the renal corpuscle; this is determined by the product of the GFR and the filterable (non-protein-bound) plasma concentration of the substance.
2. The amount of the ionized form secreted actively by the proximal tubules; this increases with increasing plasma concentration until the T_m for that substance is reached.
3. The amount of the nonionized form passively reabsorbed or secreted; this reflects the urine flow rate, the pK of the substance, and the pH of the urine.

Because so many medically used drugs are weak organic acids and bases, all these factors have important clinical implications. For example, if one wishes to enhance the excretion of a drug that is a weak acid, one attempts to alkalinize the urine. In contrast, acidification of the urine is desirable if one wishes to prevent excretion of the drug. Of course, exactly the opposite applies to weak organic bases. Increasing the urine flow increases the excretion of both weak acids and bases. Finally, excretion can be reduced by giving another drug that interferes with any active proximal secretory pathway for the drug.

Study questions: 28 to 32

NOTES

[1] Such marked transtubular concentration gradients can be established for these organic nutrients because there is only a modest "leak" of the molecules from the interstitial fluid back into the lumen across the tight junctions between cells. The statement made in a previous chapter that the proximal tubule is "leaky" and, hence, unable to achieve large concentration gradients concerned inorganic ions, not organic solutes.

[2] Movement across the basolateral membrane from cell into interstitium is by facilitated diffusion. For discussion of these mechanisms, see Guggino and Guggino, and Zelikovic and Chesney in Suggested Readings. Also, for some amino acids, "uphill" transport from interstitial fluid into cell, i.e., in the direction opposite to the reabsorptive movement, has been demonstrated. Presence of this basolateral carrier explains why, under certain circumstances, net *secretion*, rather than net *reabsorption*, of these amino acids occurs. The physiological significance of these carriers is that they supply amino acids for the cell's own metabolic requirements. (See Silbernagl in Suggested Readings.)

[3] Whether transport of urea in several tubular segments also involves active transport remains controversial. (See Marsh and Knepper in Suggested Readings).

[4] There is actually some secretion of urea into the thin limbs of Henle's loop. The source of this secreted urea is urea reabsorbed from the inner medullary collecting duct. Thus some urea simply recycles between the collecting duct and loop but does not contribute to urea excretion. (See Marsh and Knepper in Suggested Readings.)

[5] In this regard the liver's metabolic transformations are frequently important; in the liver, many foreign (and endogenous) substances are conjugated with either glucuronate or sulfate, and these two types of conjugates are actively transported by the organic-anion secretory pathway.

[6] For the specific mechanisms of urate secretion and reabsorption, see Wortman in Suggested Readings.

BASIC RENAL PROCESSES FOR SODIUM, CHLORIDE, AND WATER

Objectives

The student constructs typical balance sheets for total-body water and total-body sodium chloride.

The student understands the basic renal processes for sodium, chloride, and water:

1 States which processes—filtration, reabsorption, and secretion—apply to the renal handling of sodium, chloride, and water
2 States the three generalizations that apply to the reabsorption of these three substances along the tubule
3 Lists the approximate percentages of the filtered load of sodium reabsorbed by the various tubular segments
4 States the active step of sodium reabsorption in all sodium-reabsorbing segments
5 Lists the mechanisms by which chloride reabsorption is linked to sodium reabsorption and the one mechanism that is not
6 Lists the approximate percentages of filtered water reabsorbed by the various tubular segments in a dehydrated person and a water-loaded person; compares and contrasts these numbers and the tubular sites to those for sodium
7 States the mechanism of water reabsorption; states the water-permeability characteristics of each tubular segment
8 States the maximal urinary osmolarity; defines obligatory water loss, and states its determinants

The student understands the integration of sodium, chloride, and water reabsorption by each tubular segment:

1 States the major substances reabsorbed with sodium in the early and the mid-to-late portions of the proximal tubule
2 Describes how an osmolarity difference is established across the proximal tubule; states the luminal sodium concentration and

osmolarity at the end of the proximal tubules; defines "isoosmotic volume reabsorption"

3 Describes the changes in the concentrations of the major ions and organic solutes along the length of the proximal tubule

4 Describes the geographic separation of sodium chloride reabsorption and water reabsorption in Henle's loop

5 States how an osmolarity difference is established across the descending limb

6 States how the ascending limb of Henle's loop functions as a diluting segment

7 Describes quantitatively water reabsorption by the distal convoluted tubule, cortical collecting duct, and medullary collecting duct; states the action of antidiuretic hormone and the tubular segments and cells on which it acts

8 Describes the countercurrent multiplier system for urine concentration; states the transport and permeability charcteristics of the descending and ascending limbs of Henle's loop, the distal convoluted tubules, and the collecting-duct system

9 Describes how urea diffusion out of the inner medullary collecting ducts contributes to urine concentrating ability

10 Describes the medullary circulation and its functioning as a countercurrent exchanger

11 Summarizes the changes in volume and osmolarity along the tubule with and without antidiuretic hormone

12 Describes the obligatory relationships between sodium and water excretion; distinguishes water diuresis from solute diuresis

A balance sheet for total-body water is given in Table 6-1. These are average values, which are subject to considerable variation. The two sources of body water are metabolically produced water, resulting largely from the oxidation of carbohydrates, and ingested water, obtained from liquids and so-called solid food (a rare steak is approximately 70 percent water). There are four sites from which water is always lost to the external environment: skin, lungs, gastrointestinal tract, and kidneys. Menstrual flow constitutes a fifth potential source of water loss in women.

The loss of water by evaporation from the cells of the skin and the lining of respiratory passageways is a continuous process, often referred to as **insensible loss** because the person is unaware of its occurrence. Additional water can be made available for evaporation from the skin by the production of sweat. Fecal water loss is normally quite small but can be severe in diarrhea. Gastrointestinal loss can also be large in vomiting.

Table 6-1 Normal Routes of Water Gain and Loss in Adults

Route	ml/day
Intake	
Drunk	1200
In food	1000
Metabolically produced	350
Total	2550
Output	
Insensible loss (skin and lungs)	900
Sweat	50
In feces	100
Urine	1500
Total	2550

Table 6-2 is a typical balance sheet for sodium and chloride. The excretion of sodium and chloride via the skin and gastrointestinal tract is normally quite small but may increase markedly during severe sweating, burns, vomiting, or diarrhea. Hemorrhage can also result in the loss of large quantities of both salt and water.

Control of the renal excretion of sodium, chloride, and water constitutes the most important mechanism for the regulation of the body content of these substances. Their excretory rates can vary over an extremely wide range. For example, some persons may ingest 20 to 25 g of sodium chloride per day, whereas a person on a low-salt diet may ingest only 0.05 g. The normal kidney can readily alter its excretion of salt over this range. Similarly, urinary water excretion can be varied physiologically from approximately 0.4 L/day to 25 L/day, depending on whether one is lost in the desert or participating in a beer-drinking contest.

OVERVIEW

Being of low molecular weight and not bound to protein, sodium, chloride, and water are all freely filterable at the renal corpuscle. They all undego considerable tubular reabsorption—usually more than 99 percent (see Table 1-3)—but

Table 6-2 Normal Routes of Sodium Chloride Intake and Loss

Route	g/day
Intake	
Food	10.5
Output	
Sweat	0.25
Feces	0.25
Urine	10.0
Total output	10.5

Table 6-3　Comparison of Sodium and Water Reabsorption along the Tubule

	Percent of filtered load reabsorbed (%)	
Tubular segment	**Sodium**	**Water**
Proximal tubule	65	65
Descending thin limb of Henle's loop	—	10
Ascending thin limb and thick ascending limb of Henle's loop	25	—
Distal convoluted tubule	5	—
Collecting-duct system	4-5	5 (during water-loading) >24 (during dehydration)

normally no tubular secretion.[1] Most renal energy utilization goes to accomplish this enormous reabsorptive task.

The major tubular mechanisms for reabsorption of these substances can be summarized by three generalizations:

1. The reabsorption of sodium is mainly an active, transcellular process.
2. The reabsorption of chloride is both passive (paracellular diffusion) and active (transcellular), but in both categories it is (with one major exception) directly or indirectly coupled to the reabsorption of sodium, and this explains why the reabsorption of the two ions is usually parallel.
3. The reabsorption of water is by diffusion (osmosis) and is secondary to reabsorption of solutes, particularly sodium and substances whose reabsorption is dependent on sodium reabsorption.

Let us look more closely at these processes individually and then integrate them in descriptions of the individual tubular segments.

Sodium Reabsorption

Table 6-3 summarizes the approximate quantitative contribution of each tubular segment to sodium reabsorption. In a person with an average American salt intake, the proximal tubule reabsorbs 65 percent of the filtered sodium, the

Fig. 6-1　The most important mechanisms of sodium and chloride reabsorption in the major tubular segments. In order to focus only on sodium and chloride, we have ignored the fates and/or sources of the other substances that participate in the various cotransporters and countertransporters. Obviously, the most important of these is the potassium that enters via the basolateral-membrane Na, K-ATPases: Some of this potassium goes back across the basolateral membrane via K,Cl cotransporters, as shown in the figure, but most goes back by diffusion through the potassium channels found in almost all tubular cells (not shown in the figure). Figures 8-1 and 10-1 will show how the principal cells and distal convoluted cells secrete some of the potassium that enters. Figure 4-3 shows what happens to the organic nutrients such as glucose. Figures in Chapter 9 will show the fates and sources of the bicarbonate and hydrogen ions. The reabsorptive movements shown traversing the tight junctions are by paracellular diffusion.

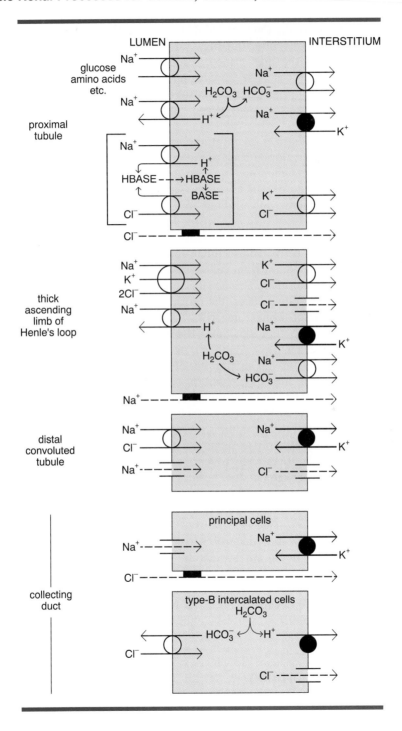

thin and thick ascending limbs of Henle's loop together 25 percent, the distal convoluted tubule and collecting-duct system together most of the remaining 10 percent, so that the final urine contains less than 1 percent of the total filtered sodium. As we shall see in Chapter 7, reabsorption in several of these tubular sites is under physiological control by neural, hormonal, and paracrine inputs so that the exact amount of sodium excreted is homeostatically regulated.

Figure 6-1 summarizes the most important specific mechanisms of sodium and chloride reabsorption in each of the major tubular segments. It may look terrifying but, in fact, when the segments are grouped together, unifying principles emerge; the figure should be used as a reference, not memorized. For the moment we will follow only sodium. We will pick up chloride in the next section.

The absolutely crucial generalization is this: In all these segments the essential event for active transcellular sodium reabsorption is the primary active transport of sodium from cell to interstitial fluid by the Na,K-ATPase pumps in the basolateral membrane (this point was emphasized earlier in Figs. 4-2 and 4-3). These pumps keep the intracellular sodium concentration very low and the inside of the cell negatively charged with respect to the lumen. Therefore, luminal sodium ions enter the cell passively, along their electrochemical gradient.

Look down the luminal membranes of Fig. 6-1 and you will see that there are various types of entry processes for sodium: Na/nutrient, phosphate, or sulfate cotransporters; Na,H countertransporters; Na,K,2Cl cotransporters; Na,Cl cotransporters; and sodium channels. Understanding how the individual tubular segments reabsorb sodium is therefore, basically a matter of knowing which entry processes apply to them. As we proceed through other chapters you will be helped automatically to learn some of these processes by knowing what else a particular segment does besides reabsorb sodium. For example, you already know from Chapter 5 that the proximal tubule reabsorbs nutrients and that the active step in this process is by cotransport with sodium across the luminal membrane.

Another generalization that arises from the last two paragraphs is that you don't have to worry about any basolateral-membrane transport processes for sodium except for the Na,K-ATPase pumps. (The function of the only other one shown in Fig. 6-1—a Na,HCO$_3$ cotransporter in the proximal tubule and ascending thick limb of Henle's loop—is to reabsorb bicarbonate, as will be described in Chapter 9.)[2]

Chloride Reabsorption

Because chloride reabsorption is mainly dependent on sodium reabsorption, the tubular locations that reabsorb chloride and the percentages of filtered chloride reabsorbed by these segments are similar to those for sodium given in the previous section.

Figure 6-2 summarizes the various ways that chloride reabsorption, whether paracellular or active transcellular, is coupled to sodium reabsorption, and Fig. 6-1 applies them to specific tubular segments.

To understand active transcellular chloride reabsorption it is necessary to recognize that the critical step for chloride in each tubular segment is from lumen to cell. The luminal-membrane process achieves a high enough intracellular chloride concentration to cause downhill chloride movement out of the cell across the basolateral membrane. Thus, luminal-membrane chloride transporters serve essentially the same active function for chloride as the basolateral-membrane Na,K-ATPase pumps do for sodium. Once again, then, you can pretty much disregard the basolateral-membrane processes (as shown in Fig. 6-1, they are K,Cl cotransporters and/or chloride channels) and focus your attention on the luminal-membrane processes for chloride. Again, I suggest that you understand the basic principles and then use this figure as a reference as needed.

Look down the luminal membranes of Fig. 6-1 and you will see that there are four of these processes: (1) a confusing-looking parallel set of Na,H and Cl/base countertransporters that we'll describe later in this chapter; (2) the Na,K,2Cl cotransporters; (3) the Na,Cl cotransporters; and (4) the Cl/bicarbonate countertransporters. The important point is that the first three of these mechanisms are dependent on sodium movement across the membrane, and are therefore linked to sodium reabsorption. Only the Cl/bicarbonate countertransporters function independently of sodium; the energy for this process is derived secondarily not from Na,K-ATPase operation but from the H-ATPase shown in Fig. 6-1. Indeed, note in Fig. 6-1 that sodium reabsorption and chloride reabsorption in the collecting duct occur in different cell types: sodium in principal cells and chloride in type-B intercalated cells.

Water Reabsorption

Water reabsorption occurs in the proximal tubule (65 percent of the filtered water), the descending thin limb of Henle's loop (10 percent), and the collecting-duct system (a few percent to > 24 percent). The first figure for the collecting-duct system applies to a maximally water-loaded person, and the second figure to a dehydrated person.

A comparison of these locations and numbers to those for sodium (Table 6-3) reveals several important points: (1) Sodium and water reabsorption occur in the proximal tubule and always to the same degree. (2) Both are also reabsorbed in Henle's loop but the limbs involved are entirely different for the two substances, and the percent of sodium reabsorbed for the loop as a whole is always greater than that of water. (3) Sodium reabsorption but not water reabsorption occurs in the distal convoluted tubule. (4) Both occur in the collecting-duct system, and the percentage of water reabsorbed may vary enormously, depending on the person's water balance. Much of this chapter will be devoted to explicating these points.

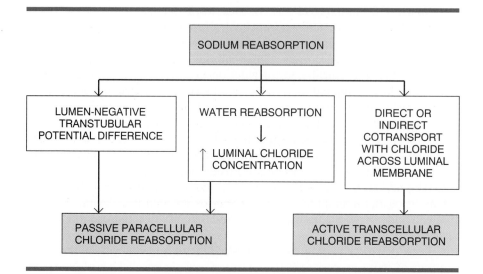

Fig. 6-2 Major mechanisms by which chloride reabsorption, whether passive or active, is coupled to sodium reabsorption. The meaning of "indirect" with regard to cotransport of sodium and chloride is described in the text; it refers to luminal-membrane parallel Na/H and Cl/Base countertransporters in the proximal tubule, as illustrated in Fig. 6-1. See text for application of all these mechanisms to specific tubular segments.

Water reabsorption occurs by simple net diffusion through the lipid bilayer and/or water channels in plasma membranes of the tubular cells and the tight junctions between the cells. The net diffusion is caused by differences in osmolarity between lumen and interstitial fluid created by the reabsorption of solutes. Recall that osmolarity is an inverse measure of water concentration—the higher the osmolarity the lower the water concentration; thus there is net diffusion of water across a water-permeable membrane from a region of low osmolarity to a region of high osmolarity.

The term "water-permeable" in the last sentence is very important—even a large osmolarity difference across a membrane cannot produce water movement if the membrane is impermeable to water. The segments of the renal tubule fall into three general categories with regard to this characteristic:[3] (1) The epithelium of the proximal tubule and descending thin limb of Henle's loop always has a very high water permeability; (2) that of the ascending limbs of Henle's loop (both thin and thick—recall from Chapter 1 that only long loops have ascending thin limbs) and the distal convoluted tubule is always relatively water-impermeable; and (3) that of the collecting-duct system can be regulated so that its water permeability is *either* very high *or* very low. These differences in water permeability explain the sites of water reabsorption given in the first paragraph of this section as well as the large range of water reabsorptions given for the collecting-duct system.

Now for an extremely important point: As we shall see, the differences in water permeabilities beyond the proximal tubule permit the kidneys to *dissociate* their reabsorption of water from that of solutes, that is, to reabsorb relatively less water than solute or vice versa. The result is that the urine osmolarity (the measure of the total concentration of solute molecules in a solution) can vary over a wide range, from extremely hypoosmotic (dilute) to extremely hyperosmotic (concentrated), compared to plasma.

The ability of the kidneys to produce hyperosmotic urine is a major determinant of one's ability to survive without water. The human kidney can produce a maximal urinary concentration of 1400 mOsm/L, almost five times the osmolarity of plasma. The sum of the urea, sulfate, phosphate, other waste products, and small number of non-waste ions excreted each day normally averages approximately 600 mOsm. Therefore, the minimal volume of water in which this mass of solute can be dissolved equals:

$$\frac{600 \text{ mOsm/day}}{1400 \text{ mOsm/day}} = 0.43 \text{ L/day}$$

This volume of urine is known as the **obligatory water loss**. It is not a fixed volume, however, but changes with different physiological states. For example, increased tissue catabolism, as during fasting or trauma, releases much solute and so increases obligatory water loss.

The obligatory water loss contributes to dehydration when a person is deprived of water intake. For example, if we could produce a urine with an osmolarity of 6000 mOsm/L, the obligatory water loss would only be 100 ml of water, and survival time would be greatly expanded. A desert rodent, the kangaroo rat, does just that. This animal never even drinks water because the water ingested in its food and produced by oxidation is ample for its needs.

To repeat, water reabsorption is driven by osmolarity differences across the epithelium of water-permeable tubular segments. Our major task, therefore, in going though the individual tubular segments is to describe how these transtubular osmolarity differences arise. In the process we will also explain how the kidneys can dissociate the reabsorption of water from that of solute in order to form a hypoosmotic or hyperosmotic urine.

INDIVIDUAL TUBULAR SEGMENTS

The important principles to be understood as we go through the individual tubular segments are how the reabsorption of sodium, chloride, and water are integrated.

Proximal Tubule

As shown in Fig. 6-1, there are several luminal entry steps involved in the active transcellular reabsorption of sodium in the proximal tubule.[4] In the early portion, a large fraction of the filtered sodium enters the cell across the luminal membrane via cotransport with organic nutrients and phosphate, the luminal concentrations of which decrease rapidly (Fig. 6-3). The rest of the sodium movement from the lumen into the cell in the early proximal tubule is mainly via countertransport with hydrogen ions. As will be described in Chapter 9, these hydrogen ions (which are supplied by carbonic acid generated from carbon dioxide) cause the secondary active reabsorption of filtered bicarbonate; therefore, in the early proximal tubule bicarbonate is the major anion reabsorbed with sodium, and luminal bicarbonate also falls markedly (Fig. 6-3). We'll come back in a minute to sodium reabsorption in the later proximal tubule.

A major fraction of chloride reabsorption in the proximal tubule is by paracellular diffusion. The concentration of chloride in Bowman's capsule is,

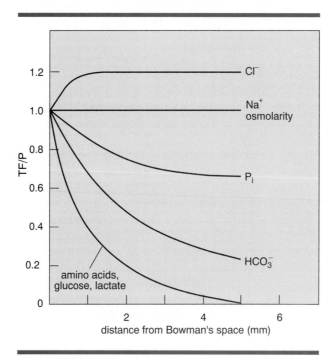

Fig. 6-3 Changes in tubular fluid composition along the proximal convoluted tubule. TF = the concentration of the substance in tubular fluid; P = its concentration in arterial plasma. Values below 1.0 indicate that relatively more of the substance than of water has been reabsorbed. Values above 1.0 indicate that relatively less of the substance than water has been reabsorbed. The concentrations of inorganic phosphate, bicarbonate, glucose, and lactate all rapidly decrease in the proximal tubule because these substances are actively reabsorbed much more rapidly than water. This is because these substances are preferentially reabsorbed with sodium in the early proximal tubule. In contrast, the concentration of chloride increases because chloride reabsorption lags behind sodium and, hence, water reabsorption in the early proximal tubule. (*Figure modified from FC Rector,* Am J Physiol *1983 249: F461, and from DA Maddox and JF Gennari,* Am J Physiol *1987 252:F573.*)

of course, essentially the same as in plasma. Along the early proximal tubule, however, the reabsorption of water, driven by reabsorption of sodium plus its cotransported solutes and bicarbonate, causes chloride concentration in the tubular lumen to increase substantially above that in the peritubular capillaries (Fig. 6-3). Then, as the fluid flows through the middle and late proximal tubule, this concentration gradient, maintained by continued water reabsorption, provides the driving force for paracellular chloride reabsorption by diffusion.[5]

There is also an important component of *active* chloride transport in the later proximal tubule, one that helps explain why sodium and chloride reabsorption are closely matched in this location. As illustrated in Fig. 6-1, it employs parallel Na/H and Cl/base countertransporters. Chloride transport into the cell is powered by the downhill countertransport of organic bases (including formate and oxalate) that arise in the cell by dissociation of their respective acids. Simultaneously, the hydrogen ions generated by the dissociation are actively transported into the lumen by Na/H countertransporters. In the lumen the hydrogen ions and organic bases recombine, and the nonpolar acid molecules then diffuse across the luminal membrane into the cell, where the entire process is repeated. Thus, the overall achievement of the parallel Na/H and Cl/Base countertransporters is the same as if the Cl and Na were simply cotransported into the cell together. Importantly, the recycling allows a small number of hydrogen ions to be involved in the reabsorption of a large number of sodium and chloride ions. It should also be recognized that the recycling and, thus, the entire system are ultimately dependent on the basolateral-membrane Na,K-ATPases to establish the gradient for sodium that powers the luminal Na/H countertransporter, without which the Cl/base countertransporter could not continue to operate. (This is why this chloride transport is termed "tertiary" active transport.)

Now for water reabsorption. As stated earlier, the proximal tubule always has a very high permeability to water. This means that very small differences in osmolarity (a few mOsm/L) will suffice to drive, by diffusion, the reabsorption of very large quantities of water, normally about 65 percent of the filtered water. This osmolarity difference is created by the reabsorption of solute. The osmolarity of the freshly filtered tubular fluid at the very beginning of the proximal tubule is, of course, essentially the same as that of plasma and interstitial fluid.[6] Then, as solute is reabsorbed from the proximal tubule, the movement of this solute out of the lumen *lowers* luminal osmolarity (i.e., raises water concentration) compared to interstitial fluid. Simultaneously, it also tends to raise the interstitial fluid osmolarity.[7] This osmotic gradient from lumen to interstitial fluid causes net diffusion of water from the lumen across the plasma membranes and/or tight junctions into the interstitial fluid.

The previous paragraph used the general term "solute" in describing how reabsorption creates an osmolarity difference between lumen and interstitial fluid. It should be clear by now, however, that we could just as well have referred simply to "sodium" since the reabsorption of virtually all solutes by the proximal tubule is dependent directly or indirectly on the reabsorption of sodium (Table 6-4). In other words, sodium and solutes whose reabsorption is

Table 6-4 Summary of Mechanisms by Which Reabsorption of Sodium Drives Reabsorption of Other Substances in the Proximal Tubule

---

Reabsorption of sodium:
1 Creates transtubular osmolarity difference, which favors reabsorption of water by osmosis; in turn water reabsorption concentrates many luminal solutes (e.g., chloride and urea), thereby favoring their reabsorption by diffusion.
2 Achieves reabsorption of many organic nutrients, phosphate, and sulfate by cotransport across the luminal membrane.
3 Achieves secretion of hydrogen ion by countertransport across the luminal membrane; these hydrogen ions are required for reabsorption of bicarbonate (as described in Chapter 9).
4 Achieves reabsorption of chloride by indirect cotransport across the luminal membrane (the parallel Na/H and Cl/Base countertransporters).

---

coupled in one way or another to sodium reabsorption constitute the overwhelming majority of all solutes reabsorbed, and so we can use *sodium reabsorption* and *total solute reabsorption* almost interchangeably in speaking of the proximal tubule.

Now we can explain the changes (really the lack of changes) in luminal sodium concentration and osmolarity along the length of the proximal tubule, as shown in Fig. 6-3. Both these parameters remain almost equal to their values in plasma; as described above, the luminal values are very slightly lower than the plasma values, but the difference is usually too small to detect experimentally. Remember that we are dealing here with *concentrations*—of sodium and total solute (osmolarity). Whereas 65 percent of the *mass* of filtered sodium and total solute has been reabsorbed by the end of the proximal tubule, so has almost the same percentage of filtered water. This is because the water permeability of the proximal tubule is so great that passive water reabsorption always keeps pace with total solute reabsorption. Therefore, the concentrations of sodium and total solute (osmolarity), as opposed to their masses, remain virtually unchanged during fluid passage through the proximal tubule. This process, therefore, is called "isoosmotic volume reabsorption."

A good example of what happens when tight coupling between proximal sodium and water reabsorption is eliminated is supplied by the phenomenon known as **osmotic diuresis**. The word *diuresis* simply means increased urine flow, and *osmotic diuresis* denotes the situation in which the increased urine flow is due to an abnormally high concentration in the glomerular filtrate of any substance that is reabsorbed incompletely or not at all by the proximal tubule. As water reabsorption begins in this segment, secondary to sodium reabsorption, the concentration of the unreabsorbed osmotic diuretic builds up and its osmotic presence retards the further reabsorption of water here (and downstream as well). Moreover, the failure of water to follow sodium causes the sodium concentration in the proximal-tubular lumen to fall below that in the interstitial fluid; this concentration difference drives a net passive diffusion of sodium across the epithelium back into the lumen (remember that the proximal tubule is a "leaky" epithelium) and so undoes a portion of the active sodium reabsorption. Thus, osmotic diuretics inhibit the reabsorption of both water and sodium (as well as other ions). Osmotic diuresis can occur in persons with uncontrolled diabetes mellitus; the filtered load of glucose exceeds the T_m for this substance, and the unreabsorbed glucose then acts as an osmotic diuretic.

Henle's Loop

As stated in the overview (Table 6-3), Henle's loop, taken as a whole, always reabsorbs proportionally more sodium and chloride (about 25 percent of the filtered loads) than water (10 percent of the filtered water). This is an important difference from the proximal tubule, which always reabsorbs water and sodium in essentially equal proportions.

Also as shown in Table 6-3, there is a geographic separation of sodium chloride reabsorption and water reabsorption. The descending limb does not reabsorb sodium or chloride, but it is quite permeable to water and reabsorbs it. In contrast, the ascending limbs (both thin and thick) reabsorb sodium and chloride, but because they are quite impermeable to water they reabsorb virtually no water. Now for a new fact: The sodium chloride reabsorption by the ascending limbs is responsible for the water reabsorption by the descending limb; i.e., the movement of sodium chloride out of the ascending limbs and into the interstitial fluid raises this fluid's osmolarity, which causes water reabsorption, by diffusion, from the water-permeable descending limb. Because the significance of this phenomenon is so tied up with events occurring beyond Henle's loop, we delay presenting the full sequence of events until we have described those segments.

What are the mechanisms of sodium and chloride reabsorption by the ascending limbs? The reabsorption of both these ions by the ascending thin limb is still poorly understood (see below) and we'll deal only with the thick ascending limb (Fig. 6-1). The major luminal entry step for sodium and chloride in this segment is via Na,K,2Cl cotransporters. The luminal membrane of this segment also has Na/H countertransporters, like those in the proximal tubule, and these provide another mechanism for sodium movement into the cell.

In addition to the *active* transcellular reabsorption of sodium a large fraction (perhaps as much as 50 percent) of total sodium reabsorption in this segment is by paracellular diffusion. There is a high paracellular conductance for sodium in the thick ascending limb, and the lumen-positive potential in this segment (described in Chapter 4) is a significant driving force for cations. (We shall see in future chapters that this paracellular pathway also applies to potassium and calcium.)

To repeat, the ascending limb of Henle's loop reabsorbs sodium chloride but not water. For this reason, it is called a **diluting segment**. Because Henle's loop as a whole has reabsorbed more solute than water, the fluid leaving the loop to enter the distal convoluted tubule is hypoosmotic (more dilute) compared to plasma.

Distal Convoluted Tubule and Collecting-Duct System

The major luminal entry step in the active reabsorption of sodium and chloride by the distal convoluted tubule is via Na,Cl cotransporters (Fig. 6-1), the characteristics of which differ significantly from the Na,K,2Cl cotransporters in the thick ascending limb of Henle's loop and so are sensitive to different drugs.[8] (Sodium channels, like those in the principal cells, also exist in the distal convoluted tubule.)

In the collecting ducts, there is a division of labor with regard to active transcellular reabsorption of sodium and chloride (Fig. 6-1). The principal cells reabsorb sodium, the luminal entry step being via sodium channels. The reabsorbing cells for chloride are the type-B intercalated cells. The "uphill" step for chloride in these cells is by a luminal-membrane Cl,HCO_3 countertransporter. There is also some chloride reabsorption in the collecting ducts by paracellular diffusion, driven by the lumen-negative electrical potential existing there (Chapter 4).

What about water reabsorption in these tubular segments? The water permeability of the distal convoluted tubule is always very low and unchanging, similar to that of the ascending limbs of Henle's loop. Accordingly, as fluid flows through the distal convoluted tubule and sodium chloride reabsorption proceeds, virtually no water is reabsorbed. The result is that the already hypoosmotic fluid entering the distal convoluted tubule from the thick ascending limb of Henle's loop becomes even more hypoosmotic. Thus, the distal convoluted tubule, like the ascending limbs of Henle's loop, functions as a diluting segment.

In contrast, the water permeability of the collecting-duct system—both the cortical and medullary portions—is subject to physiological control by a hormone (see below) and can be very low or very high. When water permeability is very low, the hypoosmotic fluid entering the collecting-duct system from the distal convoluted tubule remains hypoosmotic as it flows along the ducts and sodium chloride reabsorption continues but is accompanied by little or no water reabsorption. The result is the excretion of a large volume of very hypoosmotic (dilute) urine. This is known as **water diuresis**.

To summarize, in water diuresis the last tubular segment to reabsorb large amounts of water is the descending limb of Henle's loop; in all later segments solute (mainly sodium chloride) reabsorption continues, but water reabsorption is minimal. Note that even when very little or no water reabsorption occurs beyond the loop of Henle the reabsorption of sodium is not retarded to any great extent. Therefore, intraluminal sodium concentration can be lowered almost to zero in these tubular segments. (What makes this possible is that these tubular segments are "tight" epithelia and so there is very little back-leakage of sodium from interstitium to tubular lumen despite the large electrochemical gradient favoring diffusion.)

What happens when the collecting-duct system's water permeability is very high instead of very low? As the hypoosmotic fluid entering the collecting-duct system from the distal convoluted tubule flows through the cortical collecting ducts, water is rapidly reabsorbed by diffusion. This is because of the large difference in osmolarity between the hypoosmotic luminal fluid and the isoosmotic (300 mOsm/L) interstitial fluid of the cortex. In essence, the cortical collecting duct is reabsorbing the large volume of water that did not accompany solute reabsorption in the ascending limbs of Henle's loop and distal convoluted tubule. In other words, the cortical collecting duct undoes the dilution carried out by the diluting segments. Once the osmolarity of the luminal fluid approaches that of the interstitial fluid, the cortical collecting duct then behaves analogously to the proximal tubule, reabsorbing approximately equivalent amounts of solute (mainly sodium chloride) and water. The result is that the tubular fluid which leaves the cortical collecting duct to enter the medullary collecting duct is isoosmotic compared to cortical plasma.

In the medullary collecting duct, solute reabsorption continues but water reabsorption, by diffusion, is even greater. In other words the tubular fluid becomes more and more hyperosmotic in its passage through the medullary collecting ducts. *The reason is that the interstitial fluid of the medulla is very hyperosmotic and this is what causes water to diffuse out of the lumen into the interstitial fluid.* The crucial question, of course, is what causes the medullary interstitial fluid to be so hyperosmotic? To answer this question we must return, as I promised we would, to a further analysis of events occurring in Henle's loops.

Before doing so, however, we must complete this discussion of water reabsorption by the collecting-duct system by describing the hormone that converts its water permeability from very low to very high. It is the posterior pituitary hormone known as **vasopressin**, or **antidiuretic hormone** (**ADH**). The first name, vasopressin, denotes the fact that this hormone can constrict arterioles and thereby increase the arterial blood pressure. The second name describes the effect of the hormone's major renal action—antidiuresis, i.e., "against a high urine volume." In the absence of ADH the water permeability of the collecting duct is very low and little if any water is reabsorbed from these segments, the result being a water diuresis. On the other hand, in the presence of high plasma concentrations of ADH, the water permeability of the collecting ducts is very great and only a very small volume of maximally hyperosmotic urine is excreted. The tubular response to ADH is not all-or-none, however, but shows graded increases as the plasma concentration of ADH is increased over a certain range, thus permitting fine adjustments of collecting-duct water permeability and, hence, water reabsorption. The control of ADH secretion will be described in Chapter 7.

ADH acts in the collecting ducts on the principal cells, the same cells that reabsorb sodium (and, as we shall see, secrete potassium). The receptors[9] for ADH are in the basolateral membrane of the principal cells, and the binding of ADH by its receptors results in the activation of adenylate cyclase, which catalyzes the intracellular production of cyclic AMP. This second messenger then induces, by a sequence of events, the migration of intracellular particle aggregates to the luminal membrane and the insertion into the membrane of protein channels through which water can diffuse.[10,11] In the absence of ADH, these channels are withdrawn from the luminal membrane by endocytosis. (The reason that altering only the luminal membrane alters the overall cell's water permeability is that the luminal membrane's water permeability is much lower than that of the basolateral membrane and is thus rate-limiting.)

URINARY CONCENTRATION: THE MEDULLARY COUNTERCURRENT MULTIPLIER SYSTEM

To repeat, urinary concentration takes place as the tubular fluid flows through the medullary collecting ducts coursing toward the renal pelvis. It is medullary interstitial hyperosmolarity that, in the presence of adequate plasma concentrations of ADH, causes water to diffuse out of the medullary collecting ducts into the interstitial fluid and thence into the medullary blood vessels. The key question for urinary concentration is therefore this: How does the medullary interstitial fluid become hyperosmotic?

The complex process that sets up this interstitial hyperosmolarity is called the **countercurrent multiplier system** and takes place in the long loops of Henle that, like the collecting ducts, extend into the medulla. In earlier sections we described the characteristics of these limbs with regard to sodium chloride and water reabsorption; let us review them, adding several new facts concerning their ionic permeabilities.

1. The descending limb of the loop does not reabsorb sodium or chloride but does reabsorb water. This tubular segment has a very high permeability to water but a low permeability to sodium and chloride.
2. Both the thin and thick ascending limbs reabsorb sodium and chloride, but because they are always quite impermeable to water they do not reabsorb water. Reabsorption of sodium and chloride together from the thick ascending limb is active (Fig. 6-1), whereas reabsorption from the ascending thin limb is passive, the mechanism being unclear. However, for simplicity, we assume initially in the following analysis that sodium chloride reabsorption by both the thin and thick ascending limbs is active; afterward, the necessary qualifications will be made. Finally, the thin and thick ascending limbs are relatively permeable to sodium and chloride.

Keeping these characteristics in mind, imagine the loop of Henle filled with a stationary column of fluid supplied by the proximal tubule. At first, the concentration everywhere would be 300 mOsm/L since fluid leaving the proximal tubule is isoosmotic to plasma.

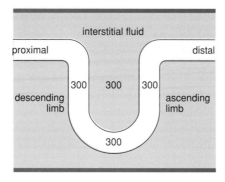

Now let the active transport systems in the ascending limbs cause the reabsorption of sodium chloride into the interstitium until a limiting gradient (say, 200 mOsm/L) is established between ascending-limb fluid and interstitium.

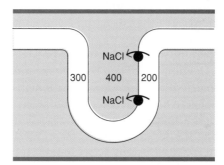

A limiting gradient is reached because the ascending limb is relatively permeable to sodium and chloride. Accordingly, passive paracellular back-flux into the lumen will ultimately counterbalance active outflux, and a steady-state limiting gradient is established.

Note that there now exists an osmolarity difference between the fluid in the descending limb (300 mOsm/L) and the adjacent interstitial fluid (400 mOsm/L). Given the great permeability of the descending limb to water, there is a net diffusion of water out of the descending limb and into the interstitum until the osmolarities are equal.[12]

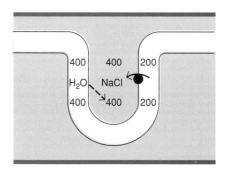

Water reabsorption by the *descending* limb occurs because of the elevated interstitial osmolarity created by sodium chloride reabsorption by the *ascending* limb. As water enters from the descending limb the interstitial osmolarity is maintained at 400 mOsm/L because of continued sodium chloride transport out of the ascending limb. Thus the osmolarities of the descending limb and interstitium are equal and both are higher than that of the ascending limb.

So far we have held the fluid stationary in the loop, but of course, it is actually flowing continuously. Let us look at what occurs under conditions of flow (Fig. 6-4), simplifying the analysis by assuming that flow and ion pumping occur in discontinuous, out-of-phase steps. Think of it as a series of freeze-frames in a movie. During the stationary phase, as described above, sodium chloride is transported out of the ascending limb to establish a gradient of 200 mOsm/L, and water diffuses out of the descending limb until descending limb and interstitium have the same osmolarity. During the flow phase, fluid leaves the loop via the distal convoluted tubule, and new fluid enters the loop from the proximal tubule. Also, there is nothing special about the numbers we have chosen for this illustration; i.e., there is nothing you know that could allow you to deduce these specific numbers.

Note in Fig. 6-4 that the intratubular fluid is progressively concentrated as it flows down the descending limb, *and that the medullary interstitial fluid is progressively concentrated to the same degree.* Although a gradient of only 200 mOsm/L is maintained across the ascending limb at any given *horizontal level* in the medulla, there is a much larger osmotic gradient from the top of the medulla to the bottom (312 mOsm/L versus 700 mOsm/L). In other words, the gradient of 200 mOsm/L established by active ion transport has been *multiplied* because of the *countercurrent* flow (i.e., flow in opposing directions through the two limbs of a loop) within the loop. It should be emphasized that the active-ion-transport mechanism within the ascending limb is the essential component of the entire system; without it, the countercurrent flow would have no effect whatsoever on concentrations.

This completes our explanation of how the medullary interstitial fluid becomes very hyperosmotic. Figure 6-5 reviews this material and that previously presented in this chapter on the distal convoluted tubule and collecting-duct system. ADH does not act on the distal convoluted tubule, and so tubular fluid remains hypoosmotic in this segment. ADH does act on the collecting ducts, and under its influence water leaves the cortical collecting duct so that the tubular fluid becomes isoosmotic to cortical plasma (300 mOsm/L) by the end of this segment. Then, as the fluid flows through the medullary collecting ducts, water diffuses out of the ducts because of the hyperosmolarity of the medullary interstitium, as created and maintained by the loop countercurrent multiplier system. By the end of the medullary collecting duct, the tubular fluid has reached essentially the same osmolarity as the interstitium. In humans, the maximal value reached in the interstitial fluid at the tip of the papilla is 1400 mOsm/L, and this is why the maximal osmolarity of the final urine is 1400 mOsm/L.

Because the osmolarity of the tubular fluid becomes greater than that of plasma only in the *medullary* collecting ducts, it is easy to forget that ADH acts

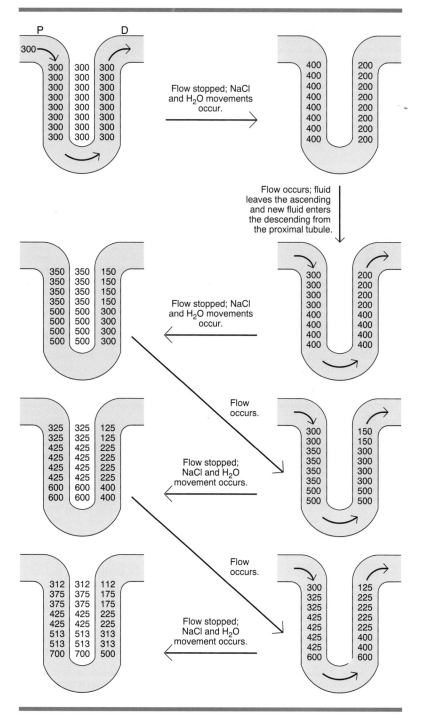

Fig. 6-4 Countercurrent multiplier system in Henle's loop. (*Redrawn from RF Pitts, Physiology of the Kidney and Body Fluids, 3d ed.; Chicago: Year Book; 1974.*)

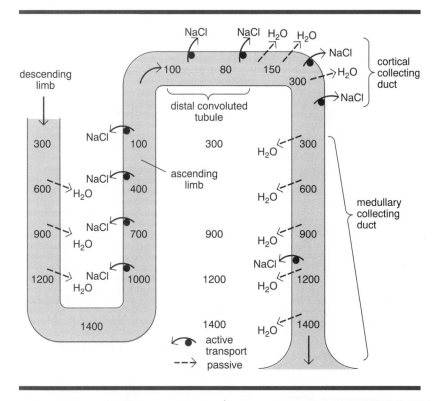

Fig. 6-5 Interactions of Henle's loop and collecting duct in formation of a concentrated urine. ADH, acting on the principal cells, increases water permeability of the collecting ducts, both cortical and medullary. Note that interstitial osmolarity at every level is identical to descending-limb and collecting-duct osmolarity. As described in the text, this figure is oversimplified in that it assumes active transport of sodium chloride by the entire ascending limb and ignores the role of urea.

not only on this segment but on the *cortical* collecting ducts as well. By permitting the reabsorption of a relatively large quantity of water in the cortical collecting duct, it causes isoosmotic fluid to be delivered to the medullary collecting duct in a volume small enough for efficient concentrating by this last tubular segment.

To reinforce further how the entire system functions, let us summarize the overall net movements of sodium chloride and water out of the tubules and into the medullary interstitium during formation of a concentrated urine. First, sodium chloride is lost from the ascending limb by active transport of sodium and chloride.[13] This sodium chloride causes net diffusion of water out of *both* the descending limb *and* the collecting ducts. In the steady state, this sodium chloride and water entering the medullary interstitium are taken up by capillaries and carried away. This is, of course, the final step during reabsorption of fluid anywhere in the tubules, and it occurs as a result of the hydraulic and oncotic forces acting across the capillary wall.

Now we must remind the reader that our model of the loop countercurrent multiplier ignored the fact that the ascending thin limb, the only portion of the ascending limb that extends into the inner medulla, does not *actively* reabsorb sodium and chloride. In this segment the movement of both ions out of the lumen into the interstitial fluid is passive, i.e., "downhill," but what establishes the gradient for this movement is not clear. Several hypotheses have been postulated during the past 20 years to answer this question, but none of them alone can presently explain all the data. The interested reader should consult the articles by Jamison and Gehrig, and Roy et al. in Suggested Readings.

The Role of Interstitial Urea in Balancing Collecting-Duct Urea

One theory proposed to explain how sodium and chloride are reabsorbed from the ascending thin limb invokes a special role for urea. This section is *not* about that hypothesized role, but rather about a quite distinct role which urea definitely does play in concentrating the urine.

From the description of the countercurrent multiplier system given thus far, one would logically (but incorrectly) assume that all the solutes in the medullary interstitial fluid are sodium and chloride. In reality, however, approximately half of the medullary osmolarity consists of urea. However, this should not really be surprising when you recall from Chapter 5 how urea is handled beyond the loop of Henle. Luminal urea concentration rises progressively along the cortical collecting ducts and the outer medullary collecting ducts as water is reabsorbed. Urea, however, is not reabsorbed because these tubular segments are impermeable to it. This high urea concentration then drives reabsorption out of the inner medullary collecting ducts, which contain a facilitated-diffusion transporter for this substance. Moreover, this urea transporter is activated by ADH. The simultaneous movement of water out of the inner medullary collecting ducts maintains a high urea concentration even as urea is being lost from these ducts.

The net result is that the urea concentration of the inner medullary interstitial fluid comes to approximate the urea concentration of the luminal fluid within adjacent inner medullary collecting ducts. In essence, then, urea *within the tubule* is balanced by urea *within the interstitium*. Therefore, the sodium and chloride within the interstitium need balance only the solutes *other than* urea in the tubular fluid. Thus, typical values for the case in which a highly concentrated urine is being formed are shown in Table 6-5. Note that if there were no urea in the interstitial fluid, the medullary interstitial osmolarity caused by sodium and chloride would have to be 1400 rather than 750, i.e., more sodium chloride would have to be transported by the ascending limbs of Henle's loop.

In this description, it is easy to lose track of an essential point: Urea, unlike the sodium and chloride reabsorbed by the ascending limbs of Henle's loop,

Table 6-5 Composition of Medullary Interstitial
Fluid and Urine During Formation of a
Concentrated Urine

Interstitial fluid at tip of medulla (mOsm/L)	Urine (mOsm/L)
Urea = 650 $Na^+ + Cl^- = 750^*$	Urea = 700 Nonurea solutes = 700 (Na^+, Cl^-, K^+, urate, creatinine, etc.)

*Some other ions (e.g., potassium) contribute, to a small
degree, to this osmolarity.

does *not* cause water to move from collecting-duct lumen to medullary interstitium. It merely balances itself. We point this out to emphasize once again
that the absolutely crucial component of the countercurrent multiplier system
is the transport of sodium chloride by the ascending loop of Henle.

Finally, because of the focus on sodium chloride in this chapter, the reader
may be surprised to discover that a maximally concentrated urine (1400
mOsm/L) may, under conditions of avid sodium chloride reabsorption, contain
virtually no sodium chloride. Much of the solute is urea, as well as creatinine,
uric acid, potassium, etc. In other words, although sodium chloride *in the
medullary interstitium* is the essential requirement for pulling water out of the
medullary collecting ducts and concentrating the urine, there need be no
sodium chloride in the urine itself.

Countercurrent Exchange: Vasa Recta

There is a unique characteristic of the medullary circulation without which the
countercurrent multiplier system could not operate, namely, the hairpin-loop
anatomy of the medullary blood vessels—the **vasa recta,** which run parallel to
the loops of Henle and medullary collecting ducts. The problem is this: What
would happen to the gradient in the medullary interstitium if the medulla were
supplied only with ordinary capillaries? As plasma having the usual osmolarity
of 300 mOsm/L entered the highly concentrated environment of the medulla,
there would be massive net diffusion of sodium chloride into the capillaries and
of water out of them. Thus, the interstitial gradient would soon be lost. But
with hairpin loops, the sequence of events shown in Fig. 6-6 occurs. Blood
enters the vessel loop at an osmolarity of 300 mOsm/L, and as it flows down
the capillary loop deeper and deeper into the medulla, sodium chloride does
indeed diffuse into, and water out of, the vessel. However, after the bend in the
loop is reached, the blood then flows up the ascending vessel loop, where the
process is almost completely reversed.

Thus, the vessel loop is acting as a so-called **countercurrent exchanger,**
which prevents the gradient from being dissipated. Note that the vessel is,
itself, completely passive; i.e., it is not *creating* the medullary gradient, only

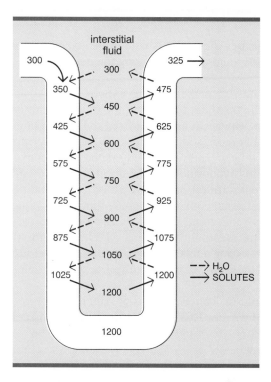

Fig. 6-6 Vasa recta as countercurrent exchangers. All movements of water and solutes shown are by diffusion. Not shown is the simultaneously occurring uptake of interstitial fluid by bulk-flow. (*Redrawn from RF Pitts,* Physiology of the Kidney and Body Fluids, *3d ed.; Chicago: Year Book; 1974.*)

protecting it. Its passive nature explains why it is called an *exchanger*. Compare its function to that of the loop of Henle, which creates the gradient and is, therefore, a *multiplier*.

Finally, it should be noted that the hairpin-loop structure of the blood vessels minimizes losses of solute or water from the interstitium by *diffusion*. It does not, though, prevent the *bulk-flow* of medullary interstitial fluid into the capillaries secondary to the usual Starling forces. By this bulk-flow process, both the salt and water entering the interstitium in equivalent amounts from the loops and collecting ducts are carried away, and the steady-state gradient is maintained.

However, the vasa recta are not perfect countercurrent exchangers, and so they do tend to carry away, as the result of diffusion, slightly more solute than water. For this reason, it is very important that the medullary blood flow is quite low compared to the cortical flow. On the other hand, it must be high enough to carry away the reabsorbed water and sodium chloride by bulk-flow, as described in the previous paragraph. Accordingly, a change in blood flow to the medulla, either too much or too little, will reduce the interstitial gradient and, hence, the maximum hyperosmolarity of the urine.[14]

SUMMARY

Figure 6-7 summarizes the previously described changes in volume and osmolarity of the tubular fluid as it flows along the nephron.

1.   Approximately 65 percent of the sodium, chloride, and water are reabsorbed in the proximal tubule, but the fluid remains isoosmotic.
2.   In the loop, water is reabsorbed from the descending limb, but proportionally much more sodium chloride is reabsorbed from the ascending limb, so that hypoosmotic fluid enters the distal convoluted tubule.
3.   Fluid remains hypoosmotic in the distal convoluted tubule, with little or no water reabsorption occurring. Thus, the ascending limbs of Henle's loop and the distal convoluted tubule function as diluting segments.
4.   Only in the collecting ducts does the presence or absence of ADH matter. With essentially no plasma ADH, very little water is reabsorbed from the collecting ducts and these segments therefore also contribute to dilution of the urine. Consequently, a very large volume of dilute urine is formed.
5.   With high plasma concentrations of ADH, water reabsorption is high in the collecting ducts. By the end of the cortical collecting ducts, the fluid

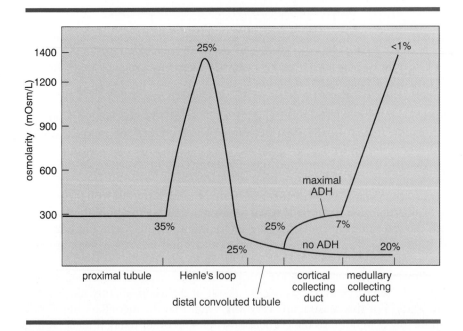

Fig. 6-7   Osmolarity of the tubular fluid and the percentage of filtered water remaining at different sites along the tubule. The latter numbers, of course, are derived simply from the numbers given in Table 6-3 for the percentage of water reabsorbed by each tubular segment.

has once more become isoosmotic to cortical plasma. Almost all the remaining water is reabsorbed in the medullary collecting ducts, and a tiny volume of highly concentrated urine is formed.

Several other points of great importance should be emphasized:

6. Large quantities of water can be excreted even though the urine is virtually free of sodium and other solutes; this, as we have seen, is a *water diuresis*, which is due to a low plasma ADH concentration.
7. Excretion of large quantities of sodium or other solutes *always* results in the excretion of large quantities of water; this is called a **solute diuresis**. This fact follows from the passive nature of water reabsorption, since water can be reabsorbed only if solute is reabsorbed first. Almost all the drugs (diuretics) used clinically to increase urine flow act by inhibiting, directly or indirectly, one or more of the transport processes mediating sodium and/or chloride reabsorption (see Appendix B for a summary of these drugs). A non-drug type of solute diuresis is *osmotic diuresis*, described earlier in the section on the proximal tubule.

Given the basic renal processes for handling sodium, chloride, and water presented in this chapter, we now turn to the mechanisms by which they are controlled so as to homeostatically regulate salt and water balance.

Study questions: 33 to 40

NOTES

[1]It is likely that under highly specialized conditions chloride can be secreted; this occurs in the distal convoluted tubule and cortical collecting duct. (See articles by Greger, and Koeppen and Stanton in Suggested Readings.)

[2]Actually, in addition to getting bicarbonate across the basolateral membrane this transporter also may contribute a small amount of active sodium transport across this membrane. If it couples 3 HCO_3 to 1 Na, as present evidence suggests, then the downhill movement of this many bicarbonates can power the uphill movement of the sodium. The contribution is very minimal, however, compared to that of the Na,K-ATPase.

[3]These three types of epithelia are typical of those found widely in nature. The differences in permeability generally represent differences in the permeabilities of the luminal membranes, which are the rate-controlling barriers (since basolateral permeability is usually always the higher of the two membranes). (See Schafer et al. in Suggested Readings.)

[4]In addition to the cotransporters and countertransporters shown for the proximal tubule in Fig. 6-1, there are also sodium channels in this segment. The quantitative contribution of these channels, however, is presently unclear. (See Palmer in Suggested Readings.)

[5]This marked reabsorption of chloride secondary to its transtubular concentration difference is largely responsible for the small lumen-positive transtubular electrical potential existing at this site. This potential causes some paracellular sodium reabsorption. However, as stated in Chapter 4, the *early* proximal tubule has a small lumen-negative transtubular potential, and this favors paracellular *secretion* of sodium. Accordingly, it is convenient to treat the average proximal potential as zero and just focus on the active transport of sodium (and the transtubular *concentration* gradient for passive chloride movement). Another reason for ignoring the passive sodium reabsorption driven by the potential in the late proximal is that if you go back far enough, you will see that this reabsorption is traceable to *active* sodium reabsorption upstream, in the earlier proximal tubule: early proximal sodium reabsorption→early proximal water reabsorption→concentration of luminal chloride→diffusion of chloride out of later proximal tubule→lumen-positive PD→passive sodium reabsorption. Finally, we have also ignored the reabsorption of both sodium and chloride by solvent drag because, as described in the next section, water reabsorption is also dependent upon active sodium reabsorpion. (For a general discussion of solvent drag and sodium reabsorption in the proximal tubule see articles by Schafer et al. and Weinstein in Suggested Readings.)

[6]The word "essentially" denotes the fact that the osmolarities of the glomerular filtrate and interstitial fluid are not exactly the same. There is a significant concentration of protein in the renal interstitial fluid, and the 1 or 2 mOsm/L difference contributed by this protein causes some water reabsorption. (See Schafer et al. in Suggested Readings.)

[7]This may not actually happen to any significant extent, however, because the interstitial space is large and because the very large blood flow through the peritubular capillaries tends to stabilize its composition. Another possible contributor to an *effective* osmolarity difference between lumen and interstitium can be understood from a consideration of the reflexion coefficients of the various solutes in the tubule, an analysis which I will not attempt here. (For a description of these factors see Schafer, and Schafer et al. in Suggested Readings.)

[8]In some species of experimental animals the Na,Cl cotransporters are not in distal convoluted tubule cells but in the cells of the next segment—the connecting tubule. The situation in human beings is not clear.

[9]The receptors acted on in the collecting duct are V_2 receptors. V_1 receptors on vascular smooth muscle mediate the vasoconstrictor effects of ADH.

[10]Such channels also exist in more proximal portions of the tubule but are not regulated by ADH. (See Verkman in Suggested Readings.)

[11]ADH indirectly exerts a local negative-feedback influence over its own effect. It induces the intramedullary synthesis and release of prostaglandins, which then oppose the action of ADH by interfering with ADH-induced generation of cyclic AMP. Accordingly, abnormal prostaglandin synthesis (either too much or too little) may account for the altered tubular responsiveness to ADH seen in certain renal diseases or during therapy with drugs that block prostaglandin synthesis. Factors other than prostaglandins also influence cell responsiveness to ADH. For example, adrenal steroids interfere in a variety of ways with ADH's action; therefore, patients with adrenal insufficiency manifest a tendency toward hyperresponsiveness to ADH.

[12]The descending limb is not completely impermeable to sodium and chloride. Accordingly, some of these ions diffuse into the loop simultaneously with water movement out of the loop. For simplicity, we shall ignore this additional complexity. (See Jamison and Gehrig, and Roy et al. in Suggested Readings.)

[13]As described earlier, sodium and chloride are also actively reabsorbed from the collecting ducts. This phenomenon helps to reduce the amount of salt lost to the urine, but it has been ignored in the balance sheet of this paragraph because it is not a very important component of the countercurrent system; i.e., its contribution of solute to the interstitium is small compared to that of the ascending limbs of Henle's loop.

[14]As described in Chapter 2, the medullary blood flow is subject to a large degree of independent control. It may well be that a major function of this control is to influence the concentrating of the urine by the countercurrent multiplier system. (See articles by Chou et al. and Pallone et al. in Suggested Readings for Chapter 2.)

CONTROL OF SODIUM AND WATER EXCRETION:
Regulation of Plasma Volume and Osmolarity

7

Objectives

The student understands the renal regulation of extracellular volume and osmolarity:

1 States the formula relating filtration, reabsorption, and excretion of sodium

2 Describes the nature and locations of receptors ("sensors") in sodium-regulating reflexes

3 Lists the efferent inputs controlling GFR and how these inputs change as a result of changes in sodium balance or fluid volumes

4 Lists the "primary inputs" controlling sodium reabsorption

5 Defines glomerulotubular balance and describes its significance

6 States the origin of aldosterone, its renal site of action, and its effect on sodium reabsorption

7 Lists the factors controlling aldosterone secretion and states which is most important for control of sodium reabsorption

8 Describes how peritubular-capillary Starling factors determine renal interstitial hydraulic pressure (RIHP) and the effect of RIHP on sodium and water reabsorption

9 Describes the direct and indirect effects of the renal sympathetic nerves and angiotensin II on sodium reabsorption

10 Lists all the effects of the renal nerves (Table 7-2)

11 Defines pressure natriuresis

12 States the origin of atrial natriuretic factor, the stimulus for its secretion, and its effects on sodium reabsorption and GFR

13 States the effect of antidiuretic hormone on sodium reabsorption

14 Lists the factors that regulate sodium excretion (Table 7-3)

15 Distinguishes between secondary and primary hyperaldosteronism; describes the hormonal changes in each and the presence or absence of "escape"

This chapter presents the mechanisms that play upon the basic renal processes for sodium and water to regulate their excretion and thereby maintain relative constancy of total-body sodium and water. As a result, as we shall see, the volume of the extracellular fluid and the osmolarity of the body fluids are also kept constant.

In normal persons, urinary sodium excretion is homeostatically increased when there is a sodium excess in the body and homeostatically decreased when there is a sodium deficit. These responses are so precise that total-body sodium normally varies by only a small percentage despite a wide range of sodium intakes and the sporadic occurrence of large losses via the skin or gastrointestinal tract.

Since sodium is freely filterable at the renal corpuscle and reabsorbed but not secreted by the tubules, the amount of sodium excreted in the final urine represents the results of two processes, glomerular filtration and tubular reabsorption:

$$\text{Sodium excretion} = \text{sodium filtered} - \text{sodium reabsorbed}$$
$$= (\text{GFR} \times P_{\text{Na}}) - \text{sodium reabsorbed}$$

It is possible, therefore, to adjust sodium excretion by controlling any of three variables—P_{Na}, GFR, and sodium reabsorption.

Plasma sodium concentration (P_{Na}) may change considerably in several pathological conditions, and these changes can influence sodium excretion by altering the filtered load of sodium. However, under most physiological situations associated with altered body sodium balance, P_{Na} changes very little

117

(except to increase transiently after a sodium-rich meal or to decrease transiently after a large quantity of sodium-free fluid is drunk) and may be disregarded as an important control point for regulation of sodium excretion. Accordingly, control is exerted mainly on the other two variables—GFR and sodium reabsorption. In general, particularly over the long term, the control of sodium reabsorption is more important than that of GFR. For example, patients with chronic marked reductions of GFR usually maintain normal sodium excretion by decreasing tubular sodium reabsorption.

The reflexes that control GFR and sodium reabsorption in response to altered bodily sodium balance are initiated by two major types of sensors: (1) extrarenal baroreceptors, like the carotid sinuses, in arteries, cardiac chambers, and great veins; and (2) the renal juxtaglomerular apparatuses, specifically the intrarenal baroreceptors and macula densa, which control the secretion of renin (Chapter 2). (The reader may be surprised that no mention has been made of sensors that might monitor plasma sodium concentration; such receptors do exist in various sites but are relatively unimportant.)

The efferent portions of these reflexes are the renal sympathetic nerves and multiple hormones, including the renin-angiotensin system and the adrenocortical hormone aldosterone. These efferent inputs act upon the renal arterioles (and glomerular mesangial cells) and the tubules. By now you should be having a feeing of *déjà vu*, for we used much of this information in Chapter 2 in describing the reflex control of renal blood flow and GFR.

It must be emphasized, however, that much control of the renal arterioles and tubules is *not reflex* at all, in the sense of utilizing neural and hormonal input arising external to the kidneys. Both GFR and tubular reabsorption are also influenced directly by the hydraulic pressure and composition of the blood (particularly its oncotic pressure) perfusing the kidneys.

Even this brief overview clearly demonstrates that the control of renal sodium excretion and, hence, total-body sodium is very much dependent upon cardiovascular pressures, acting both as stimuli for reflexes and directly on the kidneys. To understand this, one must appreciate the relationship between body sodium, extracellular and plasma volumes, and cardiovascular pressures, as summarized in Fig. 7-1. (1) Because sodium is essentially an extracellular solute (it is effectively excluded from cells by active transport), changes in total-body sodium are accompanied by essentially identical changes in the amount of sodium in the extracellular fluid. Moreover, because sodium and its associated anions account for more than 90 percent of all osmotically active extracellular solutes, the amount of sodium in the extracellular fluid is the major determinant of the extracellular *volume*. These two sentences together explain why, as stated in the first paragraph of this chapter, renal regulation of total-body sodium simultaneously achieves regulation of extracellular volume. The story is continued in Fig. 7-1: (2) Since extracellular volume comprises plasma volume and interstitial volume, plasma volume also normally changes in the same direction as total-body sodium. (3) Plasma volume, as a major component of total blood volume, is a major determinant of cardiovascular pressures. Thus, low total-

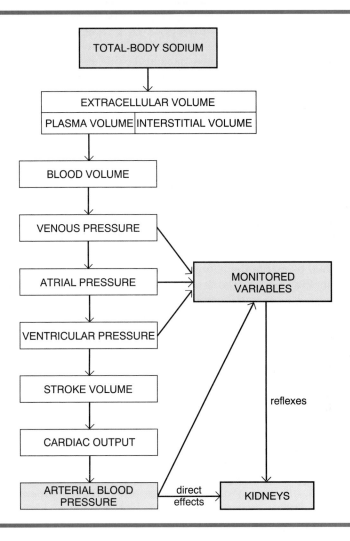

Fig. 7-1 Flow sheet demonstrating the series of derivative variables dependent on total-body sodium. In no case is any step in the sequence totally dependent on the previous one, for other factors are also involved. The major aim of the figure is to demonstrate how a change in body sodium will normally result in reductions in cardiovascular pressures that, via reflexes initiated by baroreceptors and by direct actions on the kidneys, influence GFR and sodium reabsorption.

body sodium causes low cardiovascular pressures, which, via reflexes initiated by baroreceptors and by direct effects on the kidneys, decrease GFR and increase sodium reabsorption; sodium excretion decreases, thereby retaining sodium in the body. Increases in total-body sodium have the reverse effects.

CONTROL OF GFR IN RESPONSE TO CHANGES IN BODY SODIUM CONTENT AND EXTRACELLULAR VOLUME

One important generalization to be made at the outset is that changes in GFR in response to relatively small changes in body sodium content and extracellular volume, caused for example by a change in salt intake, are usually quite small and may not occur at all. For purposes of illustration in this section, however, we'll assume that the change in body sodium content and extracellular volume is large enough to elicit a GFR change.

The *reflex* control of GFR is mediated mainly by the renal sympathetic nerves and angiotensin II. (As described below, antidiuretic hormone and a hormone called atrial natriuretic factor can also play significant physiological roles under certain circumstances.) These reflexes and the detailed mechanisms by which they lower GFR have already been described in Chapter 2. Figure 2-6 summarizes the mechanisms by which increased activity of the sympathetic nerves and angiotensin II reduce GFR. How the nerves are reflexly activated by extrarenal baroreceptors when plasma volume is reduced is illustrated in Fig. 2-7, and how renin secretion and, hence, angiotensin II concentration are increased is shown in Figs. 2-8 to 2-10.

For further review, Fig. 7-2 provides another example of how the sympathetic nerves and angiotensin II are reflexly increased by a decrease in plasma volume, due in this case to diarrhea, and produce a small decrease in GFR. By these reflexes the amount of sodium filtered and, hence, the amount excreted is reduced and further loss from the body is minimized.

At the other end of the spectrum, renal sympathetic nerve activity and renin secretion are reflexly decreased when plasma volume is increased physiologically. However, in a person ingesting the usual American diet, which contains relatively large amounts of sodium, the magnitude of these neuroendocrine inputs is already so low that a further decrease has little or no effect on GFR (or RBF).

Figure 7-2 also illustrates the *nonreflex* reduction of GFR caused by the *direct* effects on the kidney of (1) the decrease in arterial pressure, and (2) the increase in arterial oncotic pressure. As described in Chapter 2, as long as the arterial pressure decrease is still within the autoregulatory range, its direct effects on GFR are generally very small. The reason that arterial oncotic pressure rises in our example is that little, if any, protein is lost ·in diarrhea fluid, and so plasma protein becomes concentrated. A similar concentration of plasma protein occurs in the fluid loss associated with severe sweating. Conversely, an increase in salt intake will increase extracellular volume and, at least transiently, lower arterial plasma protein concentration. The result is lowered arterial oncotic pressure and increased GFR.[1]

CONTROL OF TUBULAR SODIUM REABSORPTION

As for GFR, the inputs to the kidneys for homeostatic control of tubular sodium reabsorption are the renal sympathetic nerves, various hormones, and

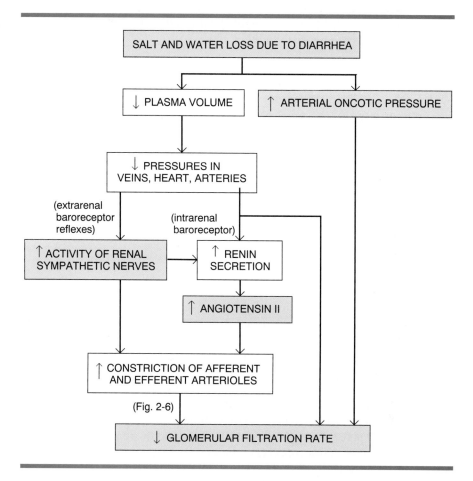

Fig. 7-2 Pathways by which the GFR is decreased when plasma volume decreases. The extrarenal baroreceptors that initiate the sympathetic reflex are located in large veins and in the walls of the heart, as well as in the carotid sinuses and aortic arch. The increased arterial oncotic pressure (due to concentration of plasma protein by the fluid loss) decreases GFR by increasing Π_{GC}. The precise mechanisms by which the arteriolar constriction caused by the sympathetic nerves and angiotensin II reduce GFR are summarized in Fig. 2-6. Renin secretion is stimulated via the intrarenal baroreceptors (decreased stretch of the granular cells) and the renal sympathetic nerves. Once the GFR has gone down, the macula densa will also participate (not shown in the figure).

the pressure and composition of the blood perfusing the kidneys (for convenience we will frequently refer to all these collectively as the "primary inputs"). The molecular effectors *ultimately* influenced by these primary inputs are mainly sodium channels and transporters in the tubular epithelial cells. The reason for the word "ultimately" in the previous sentence is that the sequences of events by which these primary inputs lead to altered tubular-cell function within the kidneys can be very complex.

1. The renal sympathetic nerves and hormones act *directly* on the tubules, but they also act indirectly, as described in the next two paragraphs.
2. Each of the primary inputs can stimulate (or inhibit) the production of one or more of the renal paracrine agents (summarized in Chapter 1, Table 1-4), almost all of which can influence sodium reabsorption.
3. Renal interstitial hydraulic pressure, as we shall see in a later section, significantly affects sodium reabsorption, and this pressure is influenced by both the primary inputs and paracrine agents.

With these basic principles in mind, we can now turn to the actual pathways that control sodium reabsorption in response to changes in bodily sodium balance.

Glomerulotubular Balance

As stated earlier, for regulation of sodium excretion the control of tubular sodium reabsorption is more important than that of GFR. One reason for this is that a change in GFR automatically induces a proportional change in the reabsorption of sodium by the proximal tubules. This phenomenon is known as **glomerulotubular balance.** (Recall that one of the mechanisms for GFR autoregulation is known as *tubuloglomerular feedback*, a name unfortunately very easy to confuse with the totally different phenomenon of glomerulotubular balance being described here.) For example, if GFR is experimentally decreased by 25 percent by tightening a clamp around the renal artery, the rate of proximal sodium reabsorption (in mmol/min) also decreases by close to 25 percent. Another way of saying this is that, in response to a primary change in GFR, the *percentage* of the filtered sodium reabsorbed proximally remains approximately constant (at around 65 percent).

It is easy to misinterpret this last sentence. It does *not* state that proximal reabsorption is *always* 65 percent of filtered sodium. It says only that *a GFR change* will not, itself, alter the percentage. There are several neuroendocrine inputs (to be described in the rest of this chapter) that act on the proximal tubule to stimulate sodium reabsorption (raise the percentage reabsorbed above 65) or inhibit sodium reabsorption (lower the percentage below 65).

The mechanisms responsible for adjusting tubular reabsorption to GFR are completely intrarenal, i.e., glomerulotubular balance requires no external neural or hormonal input; indeed, the presence of such input usually obscures the existence of glomerulotubular balance, as described in the previous paragraph. One of the mechanisms for glomerulotubular balance is explained by the fact that much sodium reabsorption in the proximal tubule is by cotransport with glucose, amino acids, and other substances; a change in GFR, of course, causes a directly proportional change in the filtered loads of these substances and thus the rate of sodium reabsorption cotransported with them.

It is unlikely, however, that this is the entire story (for other possible mechanisms see Wilcox et al. in Suggested Readings.)

To repeat, the net effect of glomerulotubular balance is to blunt the ability of GFR changes per se to produce large changes in sodium excretion. For several reasons, however, it is incorrect to assume that because of glomerulotubular balance sodium excretion is *completely* unaffected by changes in GFR. First, even if glomerulotubular balance were perfect, i.e., if the changes in GFR and absolute sodium reabsorption were exactly proportional, the absolute amounts of sodium leaving the proximal tubule would still change slightly when GFR changes. This can be seen in the example given in Table 7-1; in this example, even though reabsorption stays fixed at 66.7 percent, the absolute amount of sodium leaving the proximal tubule rises when GFR is increased and falls when GFR is decreased. Second, glomerulotubular balance is not really perfect, i.e., the changes in GFR and reabsorption are not usually exactly proportional. Thus, the proper conclusion is that changes in the GFR per se *do* cause changes in sodium excretion, but the changes are greatly mitigated by glomerulotubular balance.

Glomerulotubular balance is really a second line of defense preventing changes in renal hemodynamics per se from causing large changes in sodium excretion. The first line of defense is autoregulation of GFR, described in Chapter 2. GFR autoregulation prevents GFR from changing too much in direct response to changes in blood pressure, and glomerulotubular balance blunts the sodium-excretion response to whatever GFR change does occur in response to altered blood pressure and other GFR-altering inputs. Thus, GFR autoregulation and glomerulotubular balance are both processes that allow major responsibility for homeostatic control of sodium excretion to reside in those primary inputs that act, independently of GFR changes, to influence tubular reabsorption of sodium.

Aldosterone

The single most important controller of sodium reabsorption is **aldosterone**, the hormone produced by the **adrenal cortex**, specifically in the cortical area known as the **zona glomerulosa**. (This last term is unfortunate because it sounds like a description of a kidney area rather than of an adrenal zone.)

Table 7-1   Effect of "Perfect" Glomerulotubular Balance on the Mass of Sodium Leaving the Proximal Tubule

GFR, L/min	P_{Na}, mmol/L	Filtered mmol/min	Reabsorbed proximally (66.7% of filtered), mmol/min	Leaving proximal, mmol/min
0.124	145	18	12	6
0.165	145	24	16	8
0.062	145	9	6	3

Aldosterone stimulates sodium reabsorption mainly by the cortical collecting duct, specifically by the principal cells, the same cells acted on by ADH.[2] An action on this late portion of the nephron is just what one would expect for a fine-tuning input, since more than 90 percent of the filtered sodium has already been reabsorbed—by the proximal tubule, ascending limb of Henle's loop, and distal convoluted tubule—by the time the filtrate reaches the collecting-duct system.

The total quantity of sodium reabsorption dependent on the influence of aldosterone is approximately 2 percent of the total filtered sodium. Thus, all other factors remaining constant, in the complete absence of aldosterone a person would excrete 2 percent of the filtered sodium, whereas in the presence of maximal plasma concentrations of aldosterone, virtually no sodium would be excreted. Two percent of the filtered sodium may, at first thought, seem small, but it is actually very large because of the huge volume of glomerular filtrate:

$$\text{Total filtered Na/day} = \text{GFR} \times P_{Na}$$
$$= 180 \text{ L/day} \times 145 \text{ mmol/L}$$
$$= 26,100 \text{ mmol/day}$$

Thus, aldosterone controls the reabsorption of $0.02 \times 26,100$ mmol/day = 522 mmol/day. In terms of sodium chloride, the form in which most sodium is ingested, this amounts to approximately 30 g NaCl per day, an amount considerably more than the average person eats. Therefore, by reflex variation of the plasma concentration of aldosterone between minimal and maximal, the excretion of sodium can be finely adjusted to the intake so that total-body sodium and extracellular volume remain constant.

(It is interesting that aldosterone also stimulates sodium transport by other epithelia in the body, namely, by sweat and salivary ducts and by the intestine. The net effect is the same as that exerted on the kidney—movement of sodium from lumen to blood. Thus, aldosterone is an all-purpose stimulator of sodium retention.)

Aldosterone exerts its effect by combining with intracellular receptors and stimulating, in the nucleus, synthesis of mRNA, which then mediates translation of specific proteins. The effects of these proteins are to increase the activity and/or number of luminal-membrane sodium channels and basolateral-membrane Na,K-ATPase pumps.[3]

Control of Aldosterone Secretion

How is aldosterone secretion controlled? There are three major direct inputs to the adrenal gland stimulating aldosterone secretion (Fig. 7-3): (1) adrenocorticotropic hormone (ACTH), (2) increased plasma potassium concentration, and (3) angiotensin II. In addition, the hormone called atrial natriuretic factor, to be discussed in a later section, *inhibits* aldosterone secretion.[4]

ACTH is the hormone from the anterior pituitary that controls secretion of the other major adrenocortical hormone, cortisol. There is no question that

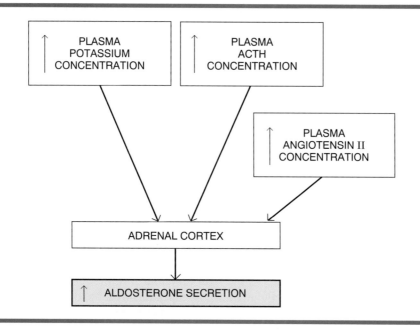

Fig. 7-3 Direct stimuli of aldosterone secretion. A reversal of all arrows in the top boxes would lead to a decrease in aldosterone secretion.

when ACTH is secreted in very large amounts, as during physical trauma, it also stimulates aldosterone secretion. Moreover, even in lower concentrations, ACTH is permissive for other stimulators of aldosterone secretion. Thus, ACTH does play significant roles in the control of aldosterone secretion. However, the secretion of ACTH is not keyed to sodium homeostasis, i.e., it does not usually participate in reflexes specifically "aimed" at maintaining a constant level of body sodium.

The influence of plasma potassium concentration on aldosterone secretion will be described in Chapter 8, in the context of the renal handling of potassium.

We are left with our third direct input, angiotensin II, as the most important stimulator of aldosterone secretion in sodium-regulating reflexes. As described in Chapter 1, the plasma concentration of angiotensin II is determined mainly by the plasma concentration of renin. Accordingly, control of aldosterone secretion in sodium-regulating reflexes is determined by those factors—the intrarenal baroreceptors, the macula densa, and the renal sympathetic nerves—that regulate renin secretion. (At this point, if necessary, the reader should review the section on control of renin secretion in Chapter 2, Figs. 2-8 through 2-10.) Thus, when plasma volume is reduced by a low-sodium diet, hemorrhage, diarrhea, etc., renin secretion is stimulated, which leads, via angiotensin II, to an increased aldosterone secretion, and this hormone then stimulates sodium reabsorption (Fig. 7-4). In contrast, when a person ingests a high-sodium diet, renin secretion is reduced, which leads via a reduced plasma angiotensin II to a decreased aldosterone secretion.

Peritubular-Capillary Starling Factors and the Role of Renal Interstitial Hydraulic Pressure

So we don't lose the forest for the trees right away, let us state the crucial generalizations first (the "forest") and then explain them (the "trees"). (1) Primary changes in peritubular-capillary Starling factors—hydraulic pressure and oncotic pressure—influence renal interstitial hydraulic pressure (RIHP). (2) An increased RIHP produced in this manner tends to reduce sodium and water reabsorption (we'll just shorten this to fluid reabsorption), mainly in the proximal tubule, and a decreased RIHP increases fluid reabsorption.

We'll analyze these two generalizations in reverse order. First, what are the mechanisms by which RIHP influences sodium and water reabsorption? For one thing, an increased RIHP causes back-leakage of reabsorbed fluid from the interstitial fluid across the tight junctions into the tubule. Thus, this effect does not alter the cellular transport mechanisms for sodium and water but rather reduces the *net* reabsorption achieved by these mechanisms, particularly in the "leaky" proximal tubule. But it is likely that an increased RIHP also inhibits the sodium-transport mechanisms themselves, either by a direct effect on the tubular cells (perhaps by altering their physical geometry) or by stimulating the release of paracrine agents that then act on the cells.

Now for the second question: How do peritubular-capillary Starling factors influence RIHP? The answer is the same as for other capillaries of the body. An *increase* in peritubular-capillary hydraulic pressure (P_{PC}) reduces the force favoring movement of interstitial fluid into the capillaries, which causes fluid to accumulate in the intersitium, thereby raising RIHP. A *decrease* in peritubular-capillary oncotic pressure (Π_{PC}) does the same thing. Thus, *RIHP is directly proportional to P_{PC} and inversely proportional to Π_{PC}.*[5]

Of course, the new question raised by this last paragraph is: What causes changes in P_{PC} and Π_{PC}? We already know the answers to this question from Chapter 2: P_{PC} is set by (1) arterial pressure and (2) the combined vascular resistances of the afferent and efferent arterioles, which determine how much of the arterial pressure is lost by the time the peritubular capillaries are reached. Π_{PC} is set by (1) arterial oncotic pressure and (2) filtration fraction (GFR/RPF), which determine how much the oncotic pressure increases from its original arterial value during passage through the glomeruli.

Teleologically, it makes good sense that P_{PC} and Π_{PC} influence RIHP and, hence, sodium reabsorption, because these phenomena are simply a logical continuation of the flow diagrams we have previously used for studying the homeostatic control of GFR. Note in Fig. 7-2 that the flow diagram initiated by fluid loss ends with three changes that then lower GFR: increased constriction of the afferent and efferent arterioles (induced by the renal nerves and angiotensin II), decreased arterial hydraulic pressure, and increased arterial

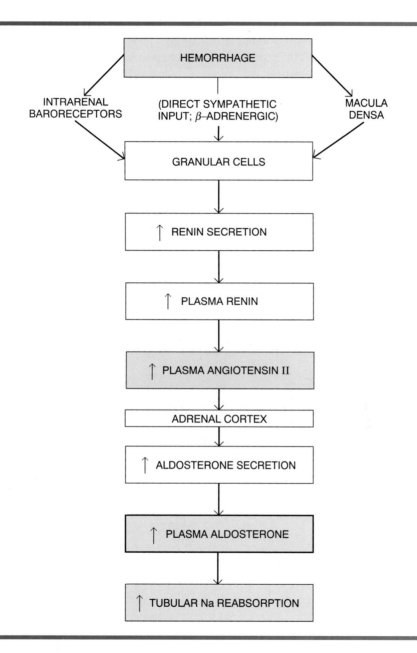

Fig. 7-4 Pathway by which aldosterone secretion is increased during hemorrhage. The detailed mechanisms by which renin secretion is stimulated during hemorrhage are summarized in Fig. 2-10.

oncotic pressure. Fig. 7-5 illustrates how these same three factors also decrease RIHP and, hence, increase sodium reabsorption. Thus, homeostatic responses that tend to lower GFR in response to a reduction in body sodium also usually increase sodium reabsorption, the "desired" homeostatic event, in response to bodily fluid depletion.

The same logic applies when the "desired" homeostatic responses are increased GFR and decreased sodium reabsorption so as to eliminate excess sodium from the body. Thus, when a high-salt diet or expansion of the extracellular volume from some other physiological cause is the primary event, there occurs: (1) decreased plasma oncotic pressure (due to dilution of plasma

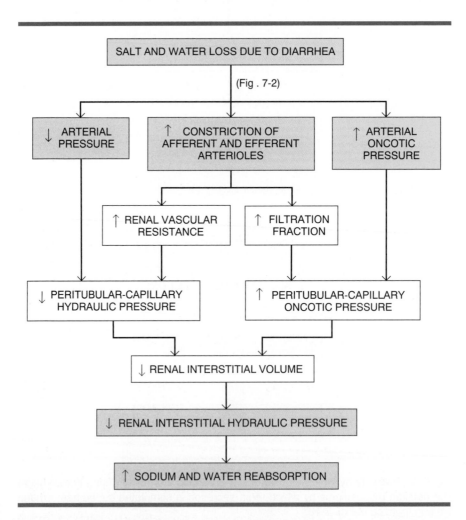

Fig. 7-5 Factors that decrease renal interstitial hydraulic pressure (RIHP) and, hence, increase sodium and water reabsorption. Compare this figure with Fig. 7-2, the figure for GFR control; the same inputs that tend to lower GFR also tend to increase sodium reabsorption via a decrease in RIHP.

proteins); (2) increased arterial pressure; (3) renal vasodilation, secondary to decreased activity of the renal sympathetic nerves and a decreased angiotensin II. (As pointed out earlier, however, this vasodilation may be very small or even nonexistent because the contribution of the renal nerves to renal vascular tone in a normal resting person is normally already so small that even complete elimination of it doesn't do much.) Simultaneously, then, the GFR goes up a small amount and so does RIHP, which reduces fluid reabsorption.[6]

Direct Tubular Effects of Renal Sympathetic Nerves

Preceding sections have detailed how the renal sympathetic nerves can stimulate sodium reabsorption *indirectly* by stimulating renin secretion (thereby leading to increased plasma aldosterone) and by decreasing renal interstitial hydraulic pressure. In addition, the renal nerves (and circulating epinephrine) also stimulate sodium reabsorption by *direct* actions on the tubular cells themselves.[7] Thus, the increased renal sympathetic-nerve activity triggered via extrarenal baroreceptor reflexes (or other signals such as fright) leads by a variety of mechanisms, summarized in Table 7-2, to increased sodium reabsorption, as well as to decreased GFR.

Direct Tubular Effects of Angiotensin II

As we have seen, angiotensin II enhances sodium reabsorption indirectly by stimulating the secretion of aldosterone and by decreasing renal interstitial hydraulic pressure. In addition, like the renal nerves, angiotensin II acts directly on the tubular cells themselves to stimulate sodium reabsorption.[8]

Table 7-2   Effects of Renal Nerve Stimulation*

1   Stimulates renin secretion via a direct action on β_1-receptors of granular cells.
2   Stimulates sodium reabsorption via a direct action on tubular cells (multiple receptors); one site affected is the proximal tubule.
3   Stimulates afferent and efferent arteriolar constriction (α-adrenergic receptors). As a result:
   a   GFR and RBF both decrease, the latter much more than the former.
   b   The increased renal resistance decreases P_{PC}, and the increased filtration (GFR/RPF) increases Π_{PC}. These changes cause renal interstitial hydraulic pressure to decrease, which stimulates sodium reabsorption, mainly in the proximal tubule.
   c   The decreased GFR and the increased proximal sodium reabsorption (effects 2 and 3b) result in decreased delivery of fluid to the macula densa, which causes increased renin secretion in addition to that of effect 1 above.

*The three categories of renal nerve effects are listed in the order in which they are elicited as the frequency of renal nerve impulses is increased to higher and higher values. Note that the direct effects on both renin secretion and sodium reabsorption occur at lower stimulation levels than those required to elicit renal vasoconstriction.

Pressure Natriuresis

I have stressed several times that the arterial blood pressure is one of the *primary* inputs acting *directly* on the kidneys to control sodium reabsorption, an increase in arterial pressure inhibiting sodium reabsorption and a decrease in pressure stimulating it. This section serves mainly to reemphasize that fact because it is so important for the regulation of arterial blood pressure; indeed, it is now thought that this relationship, by influencing plasma volume, may be the single most important long-term regulator of arterial blood pressure.

When renal arterial pressure is increased even to a small extent the kidneys show a marked and rapid increase in sodium (and water) excretion with only little, if any, change in GFR (because of GFR autoregulation); this is known as **pressure natriuresis.** The major mechanisms of pressure natriuresis are completely intrarenal. From the previous sections of this chapter, you should be able to list three possible contributing intrarenal mechanisms brought into play by the increased pressure: (1) inhibition of renin release, with loss of angiotensin II's tonic paracrine stimulation of sodium reabsorption; (2) increased production of renal paracrine agents that inhibit sodium reabsorption;[9] (3) increase in renal interstitial hydraulic pressure. Present evidence indicates that all three mechanisms are involved.[10]

Atrial Natriuretic Factor (ANF)

Many of the cells in the cardiac atria secrete a peptide hormone called **atrial natriuretic factor**, **ANF** (other commonly used names for this hormone include atrial natriuretic hormone, atrial natriuretic peptide, atriopeptin, and auriculin). ANF acts directly on the inner medullary collecting ducts to inhibit sodium rebsorption.[11] In addition, an increase in this hormone can result in inhibition of sodium reabsorption in other segments by *indirect* mechanisms,[12] including the inhibition of several steps in the renin-angiotensin-aldosterone pathway (Fig. 7-6): It inhibits the secretion of renin, and it acts directly on the adrenal cortex to inhibit angiotensin-induced aldosterone secretion. Finally, ANF, by its effects on the renal arterioles (see Chapter 2, Table 2-3) can also cause an increase in GFR,[13] and this contributes to the increased sodium excretion produced by this hormone.

The major stimulus for increased secretion of ANF is distention of the atria, which occurs during plasma volume expansion. This is probably the stimulus for the increased ANF that occurs in persons on a high-salt diet (Fig. 7-6). Although most experts assume that ANF plays a physiological role in the regulation of sodium excretion in this and other situations in which plasma volume is expanded, it is not presently possible to quantitate its contribution.[14]

Antidiuretic Hormone

As we have seen, the major function of ADH is to increase the permeability of the cortical and medullary collecting ducts to water, thereby decreasing the excretion of water. In addition to this effect, ADH also increases sodium

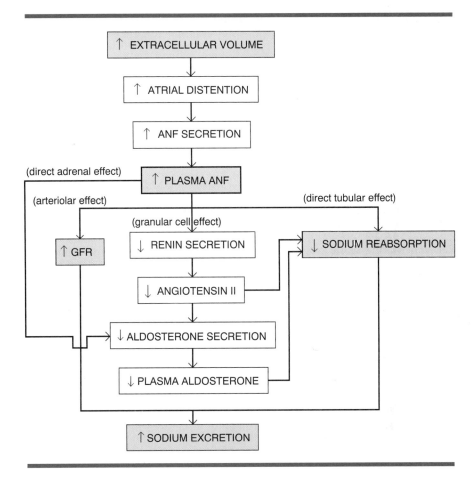

Fig. 7-6 Major effects of atrial natriuretic factor (ANF) leading to an increase in sodium excretion. The decreased sodium reabsorption caused by ANF includes not only a direct effect of this hormone on the tubules but several indirect effects, including those due to decreased concentrations of angiotensin II and aldosterone.

reabsorption by the cortical collecting duct, the same segment influenced by aldosterone.[15] This effect is particularly evident when plasma aldosterone is elevated, and ADH's action seems to synergize with that of this steroid hormone. This makes teleological sense since, as we shall see in a later section, the secretion of ADH, like that of aldosterone, is stimulated when plasma volume is reduced.

Other Hormones

ANF is not the only substance suspected of functioning as a physiological natriuretic hormone. Hypothalamic extracts contain a low-molecular-weight substance that can inhibit Na,K-ATPase in the renal tubules (and other tissues), and this substance has been found in the blood in some situations associated with expansion of plasma fluid volume. Whether it really participates in the normal regulation of sodium excretion, however, is unknown.

Many well-known hormones are able to influence sodium reabsorption. Cortisol, estrogen, growth hormone, thyroid hormone, and insulin all enhance sodium reabsorption, whereas glucagon, progesterone, and parathyroid hormone all decrease it. When the level of any of these hormones is elevated (as, for example, of estrogen during pregnancy), it will exert a significant influence on sodium reabsorption and, thereby, excretion. However, the secretion of these hormones, unlike the hormones described in earlier sections, is not reflexly controlled specifically for the homeostatic regulation of sodium balance.[16]

SUMMARY OF THE CONTROL OF SODIUM EXCRETION

The control of sodium excretion depends on the control of two variables of renal function, the GFR and the rate of sodium reabsorption (Table 7-3). The latter is controlled mainly by the renin-angiotensin-aldosterone hormonal system, the renal sympathetic nerves, the effects of arterial blood pressure on the kidneys, and atrial natriuretic factor. The renal interstitial hydraulic pressure and several renal paracrine agents play important roles in mediating some of these inputs.

There is great flexibility in such a multifactor system. Thus, for example, although the renal sympathetic nerves influence GFR, renin secretion, renal interstitial hydraulic pressure, and the tubular cells themselves, a transplanted and, therefore, denervated kidney maintains sodium homeostasis quite well because of the other known (and, probably, unknown) nonneural factors involved. Overall, the one input whose absence causes the greatest difficulty in sodium regulation is aldosterone.

In normal persons, the mechanisms for regulating sodium excretion are so precise that sodium balance does not vary by more than a small percentage

Table 7-3   Changes in These Factors Influence Sodium Excretion in Response to Changes in Plasma Volume

Filtration of sodium
  GFR
  Plasma sodium concentration (of minor importance except in severe disorders)
Tubular reabsorption of sodium
  GFR (glomerotubular balance)
  Aldosterone
  Peritubular capillary factors, acting via renal interstitial hydraulic pressure (RIHP)
  Renal nerves (direct tubular effects and indirect effects via angiotensin II and RIHP)
  Angiotensin II (direct tubular effects and indirect effect via RIHP)
  Arterial blood pressure (pressure natriuresis)
  Atrial natriuretic factor
  Antidiuretic hormone
  ? Hypothalamic natriuretic factor

despite marked changes in dietary intake or losses caused by sweating, vomiting, diarrhea, hemorrhage, or burns.

Abnormal Sodium Retention

In several types of disease sodium balance becomes deranged by the failure of the kidneys to excrete sodium normally. Sodium excretion may fall virtually to zero and remain there despite continued sodium ingestion, and the person retains large quantities of sodium and water, leading to abnormal expansion of extracellular fluid and formation of edema. An important example of this phenomenon is **congestive heart failure**. A patient with a failing heart (i.e., a heart whose contractility is too low to maintain the cardiac output required for the body's metabolic requirements) usually manifests decreased GFR and increased activities of the renin-angiotensin-aldosterone system and renal sympathetic nerves. In addition, renal filtration fraction is almost always increased—a situation that causes decreased renal interstitial hydraulic pressure. All these contribute to the almost complete reabsorption of sodium. (There is at least one factor that opposes this reabsorption—ANF—the plasma concentration of which is increased by the atrial distention of congestive heart failure.)

Why do these sodium-retaining reflexes continue to be elicited despite the fact that the person with heart failure is in markedly positive and progressively increasing sodium balance? The answer stems from the fact, described earlier, that extracellular volume itself is not *directly* monitored. In the normal person, there is no discrepancy between changes in total-body sodium, extracellular volume, and plasma volume, on the one hand, and cardiovascular pressures on the other. In other words, a reflex triggered by a change in cardiovascular pressures will end up homeostatically regulating body sodium and extracellular volume. In contrast, in heart failure, there is a discontinuity between these two groups of variables; specifically, the person has a lower than normal cardiac output and hence a lower arterial pressure at any given plasma and extracellular volume. The arterial baroreceptors reduce their firing rates because of the decrease in mean and pulsatile arterial pressure,[17] and this initiates sodium-retaining reflexes just as would occur in a normal person whose cardiac output had been reduced because of hemorrhage or severe diarrhea.

There are several other conditions, for example the liver disease cirrhosis, and the kidney syndrome nephrosis, that tend to produce sodium retention of this kind. They, too, are characterized by persistent sodium-retaining reflexes (decreased GFR, increased aldosterone, etc.) despite progressive overexpansion of extracellular fluid and formation of edema, as in congestive heart failure. All these edematous conditions, including congestive heart failure, are sometimes termed diseases of **secondary hyperaldosteronism** because they are usually associated with increased secretion of aldosterone *secondary* to increased angiotensin II, which in turn is due to the inappropriate reflexes just described.

At one time it was thought that the elevated aldosterone was sufficient in itself to cause progressive accumulation of sodium. It is now recognized that such is not the case and that one or more of the other factors that influence sodium excretion must also be operating to maintain the retention. This is nicely illustrated by the difference in sodium handling between **primary hyperaldosteronism** and the diseases of secondary hyperaldosteronism. Primary hyperaldosteronism is characterized by persistent oversecretion of aldosterone because of a primary adrenal defect, usually an aldosterone-producing tumor. Because of the increased aldosterone, sodium retention occurs initially, but after a few days, there occurs an "escape" from the effects of aldosterone, i.e., a return to normal sodium excretion despite the continued presence of increased aldosterone. After balance is reestablished, however, a persistent, small positive sodium balance still remains. What has happened is that the initial sodium retention causes expansion of extracellular volume and total-body sodium, which then initiates sodium-losing responses: (1) GFR often rises; and (2) multiple factors—decreased renal sympathetic activity, decreased angiotensin II concentration, increased arterial blood pressure, increased renal interstitial hydraulic pressure, and increased ANF—act to reduce sodium reabsorption. The net effect of these responses is to compensate for aldosterone-induced hyperreabsorption, and so sodium excretion is restored to normal.

In other words, persistent, progressive sodium retention cannot be induced by an abnormality in only one of the factors controlling sodium excretion, since opposing changes in the other factors will restore normal sodium excretion. Only when many inputs are altering sodium excretion, either appropriately, as in sodium depletion, or inappropriately, as in the diseases of secondary hyperaldosteronism, will sodium excretion remain continuously near zero. In these latter diseases, "escape" does not occur from the effects of persistently elevated aldosterone.

A variety of drugs, collectively called **diuretics**, are used in congestive heart failure and other situations to enhance sodium and water excretion by blocking sodium reabsorption. A table summarizing their mechanisms of actions is given in Appendix B and provides a nice review not only of sodium reabsorptive mechanisms but also of the interplay among the renal handling of sodium, potassium, and hydrogen ion.

CONTROL OF WATER EXCRETION

Water excretion, like sodium excretion, is the difference between the volume of water filtered (the GFR) and the volume reabsorbed. Accordingly, the baroreceptor-initiated GFR-controlling reflexes described earlier in this chapter tend to have the same effects on water excretion as on sodium excretion. As in the case of sodium, however, the major regulated determinant of water excretion is not GFR, but instead the rate of water reabsorption. As we have seen, this rate is determined mainly by ADH, which increases the water permeability of the collecting ducts, thereby increasing water reabsorption and, hence, decreasing water excretion. Accordingly, total-body water is regulated mainly by reflexes that alter the secretion of this hormone.

ADH is a peptide produced by a discrete group of hypothalamic neurons whose cell bodies are located in the supraoptic and paraventricular nuclei, and whose axons terminate in the posterior pituitary, from which ADH is released into the blood. The most important of the inputs to these neurons are from cardiovascular baroreceptors and osmoreceptors.

Baroreceptor Control of ADH Secretion

We have seen that a decreased extracellular volume, due say to diarrhea or hemorrhage, reflexly calls forth an increased aldosterone secretion. Now we see that it also induces increased ADH secretion. The reflex is mediated by neural input to the ADH-secreting neurons from venous, cardiac, and arterial baroreceptors.[18]

Decreased cardiovascular pressures cause less firing by the baroreceptors. Via afferent neurons from the baroreceptors and ascending pathways to the hypothalamus, this decreased baroreceptor firing causes stimulation of ADH secretion. Conversely, the baroreceptors are stimulated by increased cardiovascular pressures, and this causes inhibition of ADH secretion. The adaptive value of these baroreceptor reflexes is to help restore extracellular volume and, hence, blood pressure (Fig. 7-7).

There is a second adaptive value to this reflex: Large decreases in plasma volume elicit, by way of the cardiovascular baroreceptors, such high concentrations of ADH—much higher than those needed to produce maximal antidiuresis—that the hormone is able to exert direct vasoconstrictor effects on arteriolar smooth muscle. The result is increased total peripheral resistance, which helps raise arterial blood pressure independently of the slower restoration of body-fluid volumes. Renal arterioles and mesangial cells also participate in this constrictor response, and so a high plasma concentration of ADH, quite apart from its effect on tubular water permeability, may promote retention of both sodium and water by lowering GFR.

Interestingly, there are several points of interaction between ADH, which mainly controls water reabsorption, and the renin-angiotensin-aldosterone system, which mainly controls sodium reabsorption. Quantitatively, these interactions are probably of minor importance, but they add a further degree of integration between these control systems, which both go up and down together when plasma volume changes. First, as we saw in the section on sodium regulation, ADH enhances the ability of aldosterone to stimulate sodium reabsorption by the cortical collecting duct. Second, angiotensin II stimulates the secretion of ADH.[19]

Finally, as should be predictable, ADH is also elevated in the diseases, like congestive heart failure, characterized by secondary hyperaldosteronism with edema. Decreased input from the arterial baroreceptors is the most likely cause.

Osmoreceptor Control of ADH Secretion

We have seen how changes in extracellular volume simultaneously elicit reflex changes in the excretion of *both* sodium and water. This is adaptive, since the

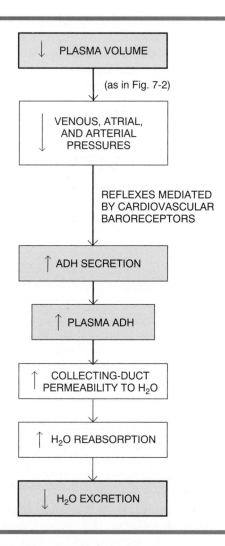

Fig. 7-7 Pathway by which ADH secretion is increased when plasma volume decreases. A reversal of all arrows in the boxes would show how ADH secretion is decreased and water excretion increased when plasma volume increases. In humans, it is not clear which baroreceptors are most important in this response. The collecting-duct cells affected by ADH are the principal cells.

situations causing extracellular volume alterations are very often associated with loss or gain of both sodium and water in approximately proportional amounts. In contrast, we shall see now that changes in total-body *water* in which no change in total-body *sodium* occurs are compensated by alterations in water excretion but not in sodium excretion.

The major change caused by water loss or gain out of proportion to sodium loss or gain is in the *osmolarity* of the body fluids. This is a key point because, under conditions of predominantly water gain or loss, the receptors that initiate the reflexes controlling ADH secretion are **osmoreceptors** in the hypothalamus, receptors responsive to changes in osmolarity.[20] The hypothalamic cells that secrete ADH receive neural input from the osmoreceptors. Via these connections, an increase in osmolarity stimulates them and increases their rate of ADH secretion. Conversely, decreased osmolarity inhibits ADH secretion (Fig. 7-8).

Take, as an example, a person drinking 1 L of sugar-free soft drink, which contains little sodium or other solute, in a short time. The excess water lowers the body-fluid osmolarity, which reflexly inhibits ADH secretion via the hypothalamic osmoreceptors. As a result, water permeability of the collecting ducts becomes very low, little or no water is reabsorbed from these segments, and a large volume of extremely dilute (hypoosmotic) urine is excreted. In this manner, the excess water is eliminated.

At the other end of the spectrum, when a pure-water deficit occurs, say because of water deprivation, the osmolarity of the body fluids is increased, ADH secretion is reflexly stimulated, water permeability of the collecting ducts is increased, water reabsorption is maximal, and a very small volume of highly concentrated (hyperosmotic) urine is excreted. By this means, relatively less of the filtered water than solute is excreted—which is equivalent to adding pure water to the body—and the body-fluid osmolarity is restored toward normal.

We have now described two different major afferent pathways controlling the ADH-secreting hypothalamic cells, one from baroreceptors and one from osmoreceptors. These hypothalamic cells are, therefore, true integrators, whose rate of activity is determined by the total synaptic input to them. Thus, a simultaneous increase in plasma volume and decrease in body-fluid osmolarity cause strong inhibition of ADH secretion. Conversely, a simultaneous decrease in plasma volume and increase in osmolarity produce very marked stimulation of ADH secretion. But what happens when baroreceptor and osmoreceptor inputs *oppose* each other, if for example, plasma volume and osmolarity are both decreased? In general, because of the greater sensitivity of the osmoreceptors, the osmoreceptor influence predominates over that of the baroreceptor when changes in osmolarity and plasma volume are small-to-moderate. However, a very large change in plasma volume will take precedence over decreased body-fluid osmolarity in influencing ADH secretion; under such conditions water is retained in excess of solute and the body fluids become hypoosmotic (for the same reason, plasma sodium decreases).

To add to the complexity, the ADH-secreting cells receive synaptic input from many other brain areas. Thus, ADH secretion and, hence, urine flow can be altered by pain, fear, and a variety of other factors, including drugs such as alcohol, which inhibits ADH release. However, this complexity should not obscure the generalization that ADH secretion is determined over the long term primarily by the states of body-fluid osmolarity and plasma volume.

The disease **diabetes insipidus**, which is different from diabetes mellitus, or sugar diabetes, illustrates what happens when the ADH system is disrupted.

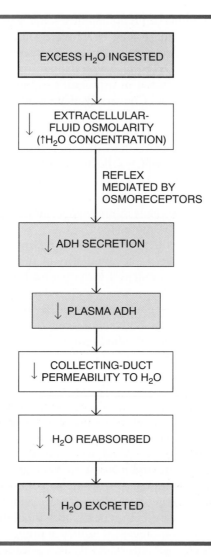

Fig. 7-8 Pathway by which ADH secretion is lowered and water excretion raised when excess water is ingested.

Diabetes insipidus is characterized by a constant water diuresis, as much as 25 L/day. In most cases, these people have lost the ability to produce ADH as a result of damage to the hypothalamus.[21] Thus, collecting-duct permeability to water is low and unchanging regardless of extracellular osmolarity or volume. In contrast, other diseases are associated with inappropriately large secretion of ADH. As is predictable, patients with these diseases manifest decreased plasma osmolarity (and sodium concentration) because of the excessive reabsorption of pure water.

This completes our description of the control of renal sodium and water excretion. Figure 7-9 summarizes the major factors known to control these processes in response to severe sweating. Sweat is a hypoosmotic solution containing mainly water, sodium, and chloride. Therefore, sweating causes both a decrease in extracellular volume and an increase in body-fluid osmolarity. The renal retention of water and sodium helps to compensate for the water and salt lost in the sweat.

THIRST AND SALT APPETITE

Now we turn to the other component of fluid balance—control of salt and water intake. It must be emphasized that large deficits of salt and water can be only partly compensated by renal conservation of these substances and that ingestion is the ultimate compensatory mechanism.

The centers that mediate thirst are located in the hypothalamus (very close to those areas that produce ADH). The subjective feeling of **thirst**, which drives one to obtain and ingest water, is stimulated both by reduced plasma volume and by increased body-fluid osmolarity. The adaptive significance of both are self-evident. Note that these are precisely the same changes that stimulate ADH production, and the receptors—osmoreceptors and cardiovascular baroreceptors—that initiate the ADH-controlling reflexes are in the same locations as those for thirst. The thirst response, however, is significantly less sensitive than is the ADH response.

There are also other pathways controlling thirst. For example, dryness of the mouth and throat causes profound thirst, which is relieved by merely moistening them. Also, when animals such as the camel (and humans, to a lesser extent) become markedly dehydrated, they will rapidly drink just enough water to replace their previous losses and then stop. What is amazing is that when they stop, the water has not yet had time to be absorbed from the gastrointestinal tract into the blood. Some kind of metering of the water intake by the gastrointestinal tract has occurred, but its nature remains a mystery.

Angiotensin II is yet another factor that stimulates thirst—by a direct effect on the brain—and this hormone constitutes one of the pathways by which thirst is stimulated when extracellular volume is decreased.

Salt appetite, which is the analogue of thirst, is also an extremely important component of sodium homeostasis in most mammals. It is clear that salt appetite in these species is innate and consists of two components: (1) *hedonistic* appetite and (2) *regulatory* appetite. In other words, (1) animals like salt and eat it whenever they can, regardless of whether they are salt-deficient, and (2) their drive to obtain salt is markedly increased in the presence of deficiency.

The significance of these animal studies for humans, however, is unclear. Salt craving does seem to occur in humans who are severely salt-depleted, but the contribution of such regulatory salt appetite to everyday sodium homeostasis in normal persons is probably slight. On the other hand, humans do seem to have a strong hedonistic appetite for salt, as manifested by almost univer-

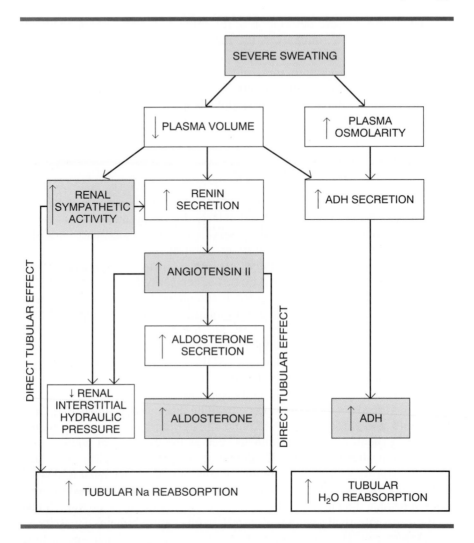

Fig. 7-9 Summary of major factors that increase tubular sodium and water reabsorption in severe sweating. (As noted in the text, ADH also enhances sodium reabsorption, but this is a relatively minor effect and is not shown in the figure.) These changes, coupled with the decrease in GFR that also occurs, homeostatically reduce urinary sodium and water loss. (To visualize the response to a high-sodium diet or the infusion of saline simply replace "severe sweating" with these events, reverse all the arrows in the boxes, and add an increase in ANF, the result of atrial distention.)

sally large intakes of sodium whenever it is cheap and readily available. Thus, the average American intake of salt is 10 to 15 g/day despite the fact that humans can survive quite normally on less than 0.5 g/day. Present evidence, although controversial, suggests that a large salt intake may be a contributor to the pathogenesis of hypertension in susceptible individuals.

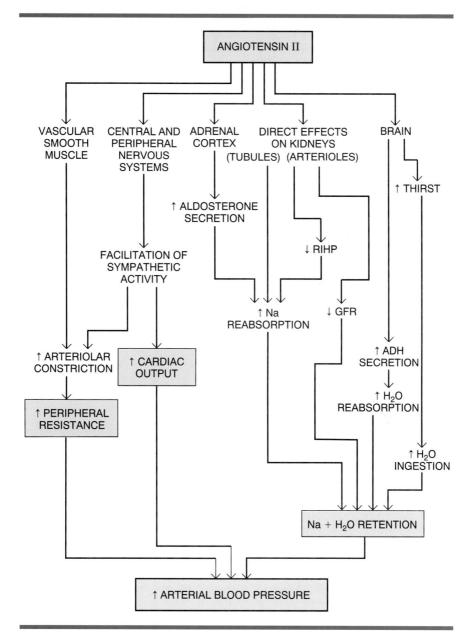

Fig. 7-10 Summary of those angiotensin-mediated actions that facilitate fluid retention and elevate the arterial blood pressure. The arrow connecting "Na and H_2O retention" to "arterial blood pressure" is a shortcut for the sake of simplicity—of course, fluid retention influences arterial blood pressure only by altering cardiac output and peripheral resistance.

SUMMARY OF THE EFFECTS OF ANGIOTENSIN II

We have presented various effects of angiotensin II in this chapter and in Chapter 2, and this is a good place to summarize them. Angiotensin II exerts a wide array of effects on many bodily sites, but the common denominator of those with which we are concerned is that they all favor both salt retention and elevation of arterial blood pressure. Figure 7-10 summarizes these effects, adding the fact, not previously mentioned, that angiotensin II, by a variety of mechanisms, facilitates the activity of the sympathetic nervous system (e.g., by increasing the amount of norepinephrine released during action potentials). It is crucial to recognize that when renin secretion is elevated in response to *physiological* stimuli, such as sodium deprivation, all the effects of angiotensin II shown in Fig. 7-10 serve to minimize fluid depletion and to prevent blood pressure from falling below normal. In contrast, when an inappropriate increase in renin secretion occurs because of disease (as in renal artery stenosis, for example), these effects will tend to elevate the blood pressure above normal.

Study questions: 41 to 56

NOTES

[1] In all the examples in this paragraph, the change in arterial-plasma oncotic pressure is in the appropriate direction to reestablish salt balance by decreasing or increasing GFR and, hence, salt excretion. This is not, however, the case for hemorrhage. Hemorrhage per se does not immediately alter plasma protein concentration, since all blood components are lost in equivalent proportions. However, the blood loss is followed by a net movement of interstitial fluid into the vascular compartment. This entry of protein-free fluid *lowers* the plasma protein concentration, and this decreased plasma oncotic pressure would tend to *raise* GFR. Thus, the various factors—increased renal sympathetic nerve activity, increased angiotensin II, and decreased arterial pressure—that successfully reduce GFR in hemorrhage are actually being opposed by a decrease in arterial-plasma oncotic pressure. This analysis is presented as a reminder that the GFR response to any given situation represents the algebraic sum of multiple forces.

[2] It is possible that aldosterone also stimulates sodium reabsorption by the thick ascending limb of Henle's loop. (See Funder in Suggested Readings.)

[3] Because aldosterone's enhancement of sodium reabsorption requires time (at least 45 min) for protein synthesis, decreases in sodium excretion that occur within minutes (as, for example, immediately upon standing up) are clearly not caused by increased aldosterone.

[4] Another direct input that inhibits aldosterone secretion is an increase in plasma osmolarity. In humans, the osmolarity stimulus is probably relatively minor, a fact that makes sense teleologically since osmolarity generally changes very little despite marked changes in extracellular *volume*. Water movements into or out of body cells tend to

keep osmolarity (and, thereby, plasma sodium concentration) relatively stable. (See Schneider in Suggested Readings for the possible physiological significance of this osmolarity-aldosterone relationship.)

[5]This discussion of the determinants of RIHP focuses entirely on peritubular-capillary factors. Of course, there is another determinant of RIHP—the rate of movement of reabsorbed fluid from the tubular lumen into the interstitium. Primary changes in the rate of this reabsorptive step will produce changes in RIHP, which will in turn exert a local negative feedback effect on the rate of reabsorption. Because this sequence is always secondary to a primary change in reabsorptive rate, we ignore it; we are really interested here only in how a primary change in RIHP causes a secondary change in reabsorptive rate, and that is why we focus only on the peritubular-capillary factors as determinants of RIHP.

[6]This section has emphasized that renal vasodilators can reduce sodium reabsorption by increasing RIHP. Another possible mechanism, not discussed in the text, by which vasoactive agents might influence sodium reabsorption is by changes in medullary blood flow. Specifically, it has been hypothesized that an increase in medullary blood flow would reduce sodium reabsorption by the ascending thin limb of Henle's loop. (See Knox and Granger in Suggested Readings.)

[7]The major site of this stimulation is the proximal tubule. The receptor type in the cells of this segment are alpha$_1$-adrenergic. However, recent evidence indicates that other tubular sites and receptor types also play a role. (See Garg in Suggested Readings.)

[8]As with the sympathetic nerves the proximal tubule is definitely a site of this direct stimulation, which is exerted mainly on the Na/H countertransporters, but other segments may also be involved. A source of potential confusion is the fact that angiotensin II, when present in extremely large ("pharmacological") amounts, acts directly on the tubule to inhibit sodium reabsorption rather than stimulate it.

[9]The natriuretic paracrine agents most implicated are PGE_2 and nitric oxide. (See Knox and Granger in Suggested Readings.)

[10]As described in note 6, another possible mechanism is increased medullary blood flow.

[11]ANF probably also acts directly on the cortical collecting duct to inhibit sodium reabsorption. The second messenger for the direct tubular effects is cGMP, and at least part of the effect is due to inhibition of luminal-membrane sodium channels.

[12]ANF also acts on the kidneys to inhibit sodium reabsorption by the proximal tubule, but in this case the tubular effect must be secondary to some other intrarenal actions since there are no receptors for the hormone on proximal tubular cells. There are probably at least three mechanisms that account for this inhibition: (1) ANF stimulates dopamine secretion by the proximal tubular cells, with the dopamine then acting back on the cells to inhibit their sodium reabsorption. (2) As stated in the text, ANF also inhibits the secretion of renin, which would result in less angiotensin II generation in the kidney; since angiotensin II stimulates proximal sodium reabsorption, the drop in intrarenal angiotensin II caused by ANF would also contribute to decreased proximal reabsorption. (3) Because of its actions on renal arterioles the hormone raises renal

interstitial hydraulic pressure, and this too would tend to reduce sodium reabsorption by the proximal tubule and other segments as well.

[13]ANF also increases glomerular K_f, probably due to dilation of glomerular mesangial cells.

[14]Some experts believe that ANF is not a physiological regulator of sodium excretion at all. (See Goetz in Suggested Readings.) Another fascinating recent finding (see this same article) is that the kidneys themselves produce a peptide, called urodilatin, which may be identical to the 126-residue prohormone of ANF, and it has been hypothesized that this peptide functions as an intrarenal natriuretic agent.

[15]In some species, but not in humans, ADH also stimulates sodium reabsorption by the thick ascending limb of Henle's loop. (See Greger in Suggested Readings for Chapter 6.)

[16]Parathyroid hormone may be an exception to this generalization. Although its secretion is controlled mainly by plasma calcium concentration, it is also increased during volume expansion and may contribute to the inhibition of proximal tubular sodium reabsorption in this situation. (See Seldin and Giebisch, in Suggested Readings.)

[17]In addition, baroreceptors in the great veins and cardiac chambers appear to be damaged by (or adapted to) the engorgement occurring in these locations and manifest decreased rates of firing despite the marked degree of distention in these areas.

[18]In non-primates, baroreceptors in the left atrium are the major volume receptors controlling ADH secretion, but the picture is presently unclear for humans. (See Robertson in Suggested Readings.)

[19]There is, however, disagreement about whether plasma concentrations of angiotensin II are ever high enough physiologically to stimulate ADH secretion. (See Robertson in Suggested Readings.)

[20]There are also osmoreceptors located in the liver and probably other sites as well. The mechanism by which the hypothalamic osmoreceptors detect changes in osmolarity is unknown. Some evidence suggests that these receptors may actually be sensitive to sodium rather than to osmolarity. The end result is the same, since sodium is normally the major determinant of osmolarity. Of clinical interest is the fact that the receptors are not affected by changes in plasma urea or glucose; accordingly, the increases in these substances in uremia and diabetes mellitus, respectively, do not increase ADH secretion. (See Robertson in Suggested Readings.)

[21]The major exception is the disease known as *nephrogenic* diabetes insipidus, in which the defect is not failure to secrete ADH but failure of the kidneys to respond to this hormone. The cause of this is genetic absence of receptors for ADH on collecting-duct cells.

RENAL REGULATION OF POTASSIUM BALANCE

8

Objectives

The student understands the internal exchanges of potassium:

1 States the normal distribution of body potassium
2 States the effects of epinephrine, insulin, acidosis, and alkalosis on potassium movement into cells

The student understands the renal regulation of potassium:

1 States the relative amounts of potassium reabsorbed by the proximal tubule and thick ascending limb of Henle's loop, regardless of the state of potassium balance
2 Contrasts the contribution of the cortical collecting duct in persons on a high- and low-potassium diet
3 Describes the mechanisms by which active potassium secretion and reabsorption are accomplished by the cortical collecting duct; states which cells are involved
4 Lists the inputs that control the rate of potassium secretion by the cortical collecting duct so as to regulate potassium balance homeostatically
5 Describes the pathway by which changes in potassium balance influence aldosterone secretion
6 Describes the relationship between potassium secretion and fluid delivery to the cortical collecting duct; explains how this relationship prevents changes in aldosterone produced by altered sodium balance from perturbing potassium secretion; states the effects of most diuretic drugs and osmotic diuretics on potassium secretion
7 States the direct action of ADH on potassium secretion, and describes how water diuresis does not cause increased potassium secretion
8 Describes the effects of alkalosis on potassium secretion and balance

The potassium concentration of the extracellular fluid is a closely regulated quantity. The importance of maintaining this concentration relatively constant stems primarily from the role of potassium in the excitability of nerve and muscle. The resting membrane potentials of these tissues are directly related to the ratio of intracellular to extracellular potassium concentration. Raising the extracellular potassium concentration lowers the resting membrane potential, thus increasing cell excitability. Conversely, lowering the extracellular potassium concentration hyperpolarizes cell membranes and reduces their excitability.

Extracellular potassium concentration is a function of two variables: (1) the total amount of potassium in the body, and (2) the distribution of this potassium between the extracellular and intracellular fluid compartments. The first variable, total-body potassium, is determined by the relative rates of potassium intake and excretion. Normal individuals remain in potassium balance, as they do in sodium balance, by excreting daily an amount of urinary potassium equal to the amount of potassium ingested minus the small amounts eliminated in the feces and sweat. Normally, potassium losses via sweat and the gastrointestinal tract are small, but very large quantities can be lost from the tract during vomiting or diarrhea. Again, the control of renal function is the major mechanism by which total-body potassium is maintained in balance.

However, before describing the renal handling of potassium, we must briefly summarize the second variable determining extracellular potassium concentration—the distribution of total-body potassium between the extracellular and intracellular fluid compartments.

REGULATION OF INTERNAL POTASSIUM DISTRIBUTION

Approximately 98 percent of total-body potassium is located within cells because of the Na, K-ATPase plasma-membrane pumps, which actively transport potassium into cells. Since the amount of potassium in the extracellular compartment is so small even very slight shifts of potassium into or out of the cells can produce large changes in extracellular potassium concentration. Such shifts, particularly in muscle, are to some extent under physiological control. Therefore, when extracellular potassium concentration changes because of changes either in total-body potassium (i.e., imbalances between intake and excretion) or internal shifts secondary to other events (cell damage, for example), potassium moves into or out of the cells, thereby minimizing the changes in extracellular concentration. The major factors involved in these homeostatic processes are epinephrine and insulin, both of which cause increased potassium uptake by muscle (and certain other cells) through stimulation of plasma-membrane Na,K-ATPase.[1]

The effect of epinephrine on potassium uptake is probably of greatest physiological importance during exercise and trauma. In these situations potassium moves *out* of the exercising muscle cells or the damaged cells, which raises extracellular potassium concentration. However, at the same time, exercise or trauma increases adrenomedullary secretion of epinephrine, and this hormone's stimulation of potassium uptake by other cells partially offsets the outflow from the exercising or damaged cells.

The rise in plasma insulin concentration after a meal plays an important role in causing the movement of the ingested and absorbed potassium into cells. This potassium then slowly comes out of cells between meals to be excreted. Moreover, a large increase in plasma potassium concentration stimulates insulin secretion at any time, and the additional insulin induces greater potassium uptake by the cells—a negative feedback system for opposing acute elevations in plasma potassium concentration.

Thus far, the discussion has dealt with factors that *homeostatically* regulate internal potassium movements to minimize changes in extracellular potassium concentration. However, other factors can influence potassium movements into or out of cells but are not homeostatic mechanisms for regulating extracellular potassium. Instead they may displace extracellular potassium concentration away from normal. The most important of these is the extracellular-fluid hydrogen-ion concentration: An increase in extracellular-fluid hydrogen-ion concentration (acidosis) is often associated with net potassium movement out of cells, whereas a decrease in extracellular-fluid hydrogen-ion concentration (alkalosis) causes net potassium movement into them.[2] It is as though potassium and hydrogen ions were "exchanging" across plasma membranes (i.e., hydrogen ions moving into the cell during acidosis and out during alkalosis, with potassium doing just the opposite), but the precise mechanism underlying these "exchanges" has not yet been clarified.

BASIC RENAL MECHANISMS

Potassium is freely filterable at the renal corpuscle. The amount of potassium excreted in the urine by a normal person eating a typical American diet is 5 to 15 percent of the filtered quantity (about 35 to 100 mmol per day). This fact establishes the existence of tubular potassium reabsorption. Indeed, when a person is eating a diet very low in potassium or is potassium-depleted, say because of gastrointestinal losses, the percentage reabsorbed can go up a good deal more, although never to as complete a level as sodium reabsorption. In contrast, with excessive dietary potassium intake or under certain other conditions (see below) excreted potassium can exceed the filtered quantity by a large amount. This fact establishes that the tubule is also capable of secreting potassium. Thus, for the entire tubule either net tubular reabsorption or net tubular secretion may occur. As we shall see, the tubular segments that account for these large differences in potassium excretion are the more distal segments.

The tubular handling of potassium is summarized in Table 8-1. *Regardless of a person's bodily potassium status* the proximal tubule reabsorbs approximately 55 percent of filtered potassium, and the thick ascending limb of

Table 8-1 Summary of Tubular Potassium Transport

	Normal- or high-potassium diet	Low-potassium diet or potassium depletion
Proximal tubule	Reabsorption (55%)*	Reabsorption (55%)
Thick ascending limb of Henle's loop	Reabsorption (30%)	Reabsorption (30%)
Distal convoluted tubule and cortical collecting duct	**Secretion**	**Reabsorption**
Medullary collecting duct	Reabsorption	Reabsorption

*The percents are in reference to the filtered load of potassium. This table disregards potassium recycling in the renal medulla (end-of-chapter note 3).

Henle's loop about 30 percent.[3] The mechanisms for potassium reabsorption in these two segments are deducible from our discussions of ion transport in other chapters: (1) Reabsorption in the proximal tubule is mainly by paracellular diffusion, the concentration gradient for which is created, as for urea and chloride, by water reabsorption.[4] (2) Reabsorption in the thick ascending limb is, like that of sodium, partially active [driven by the luminal-membrane Na,K,2 Cl cotransporter (Fig. 6-1)][5] and partially by paracellular diffusion, driven by the lumen-positive transtubular potential difference in this segment. Thus, potassium reabsorption by both segments is ultimately dependent upon sodium reabsorption.

What about the rest of the tubule (Table 8-1)? For a person who is on a low-potassium diet or is potassium-depleted for some other reason, the distal segments reabsorb potassium. The end result is that only a very small amount of potassium is excreted.

In contrast, for a person on a normal- or high-potassium diet, the distal convoluted tubule and the cortical collecting duct both manifest net potassium secretion, and the amount of potassium in the tubule increases markedly. The greater the person's potassium intake or positive bodily-potassium balance, the greater the amount of potassium secreted by these segments. (The final tubular segment, the medullary collecting duct, still usually reabsorbs potassium.[6]) The overall result, therefore, of the various tubular contributions in persons on a normal- or high-potassium diet is that *the great majority of the excreted potassium is potassium that was secreted by the distal convoluted tubule and cortical collecting duct.*

Because the contribution (either reabsorptive or secretory) of the cortical collecting duct is much greater than that of the distal convoluted tubule, we shall for simplicity refer only to it in the remainder of this chapter. How is it that the cortical collecting duct can manifest either net reabsorption or net secretion? Recall once again that the collecting-duct system contains principal cells and intercalated cells. It is the principal cells—the same cells we described earlier as the aldosterone-regulated reabsorbers of sodium and the ADH-regulated reabsorbers of water—that secrete potassium. In contrast, the intercalated cells—specifically those of the A type—reabsorb potassium. (This reabsorptive process also mediates the simultaneous tubular secretion of hydrogen ions and will be described in Chapter 9.) Under conditions of normal- or positive-potassium balance, principal-cell potassium secretion is much greater than potassium reabsorption by the type-A intercalated cells, and so the cortical collecting duct shows net secretion. During potassium depletion, however, the principal cells cease their secretion, and so net reabsorption becomes manifest.

Thus, the renal handling of potassium may be summarized by the following important generalization (Table 8-1): *Differences in potassium excretion over the usual physiological range are due primarily to differences in the amount of potassium secreted by the cortical collecting duct.* It is this variable that is controlled to regulate homeostatically urinary potassium excretion. There is little, if any, homeostatic control over potassium reabsorption in any tubular segment.[7]

So dominant is this secretory process in determining changes in potassium excretion that in describing the control of potassium excretion we will tend to ignore any contribution of changes in either filtered potassium (GFR $\times P_K$) or tubular transport proximal to the collecting-duct system. It must be pointed out, however, that under certain conditions, potassium reabsorption in the proximal tubule and/or Henle's loop may be decreased and that a large quantity of the potassium excreted may represent filtered potassium that has not been reabsorbed. For example, diuretics that inhibit sodium reabsorption by the proximal tubule or thick ascending limb of Henle's loop also inhibit potassium reabsorption at these sites; the reasons should be clear from the sodium-dependence of potassium reabsorption by these segments. Osmotic diuretics, as should also be predictable, interfere with potassium reabsorption by these segments, and this is one reason for the marked urinary loss of potassium suffered by patients with uncontrolled diabetes mellitus (another will be given below).

MECHANISM OF POTASSIUM SECRETION IN THE CORTICAL COLLECTING DUCT

To restate our generalization: Differences in potassium excretion over the usual physiological range are due primarily to differences in the amount of potassium secreted by the principal cells of the cortical collecting duct. Figure 8-1 summarizes the pathway for potassium secretion in these cells.

This secretion involves active transport of potassium into the cell across the basolateral membrane and passive exit across the luminal membrane. The critical event is the active transport of potassium from interstitial fluid across the basolateral membrane into the cell. This active transport step, which is mediated via Na,K-ATPase pumps, creates a high intracellular potassium con-

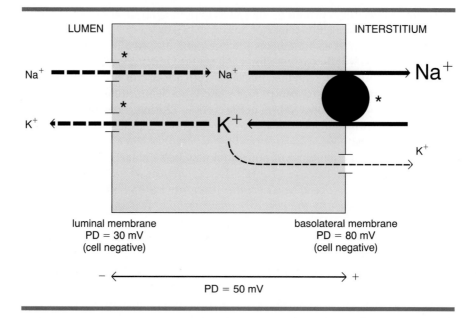

Fig. 8-1 Model of transcellular potassium secretion by principal cells of the cortical collecting duct. This figure is essentially the same as Fig. 4-2 and the principal cell in Fig. 6-1, which were used to demonstrate sodium reabsorption, the only addition being the crucial one of potassium channels in the luminal membrane. Potassium is actively moved into the cell by the basolateral-membrane Na,K-ATPase pumps and then diffuses across the luminal membrane through these potassium channels. Note that there is also some potassium diffusion back across the basolateral-membrane channels from the cell into the interstitial fluid; this is "wasted" potassium so far as potassium secretion is concerned. The amount is small, however, compared to movement through the luminal-membrane potassium channels because of the differences in electrical potentials across the two membranes and the much smaller number of potassium channels in the basolateral membrane. [Also, in addition to the luminal-membrane potassium channels there are some luminal-membrane K,Cl cotransporters (not shown in the figure), which transport additional potassium into the lumen.] Both the reabsorption of sodium and secretion of potassium by these cells are regulated by aldosterone, and the asterisks indicate the processes controlled by this hormone.

centration so that there is a concentration gradient favoring net potassium diffusion from cell into lumen through the numerous luminal potassium channels in this tubular segment.[8] [Note, however, that the potassium concentration gradient across the luminal membrane is opposed by an electrical force (30 mV, cell-negative) that favors net diffusion from lumen to cell; however, this opposing electrical force is not as large as the chemical force (the concentration gradient), and so the total electrochemical gradient favors net diffusion of potassium into the lumen.[9]]

HOMEOSTATIC CONTROL OF POTASSIUM SECRETION BY THE CORTICAL COLLECTING DUCT

What are the factors that influence potassium secretion by the principal cells of the cortical collecting duct to achieve homeostasis of bodily potassium? The single most important factor is as follows: When a high-potassium diet is ingested (Fig. 8-2), plasma potassium concentration increases, although very slightly, and this drives enhanced basolateral uptake via the basolateral Na,K-ATPase pumps. The resulting increase in intracellular potassium concentration enhances the gradient for potassium movement into the lumen and raises potassium secretion. Conversely, a low-potassium diet or a negative-potassium balance, e.g., from diarrhea, lowers potassium concentration

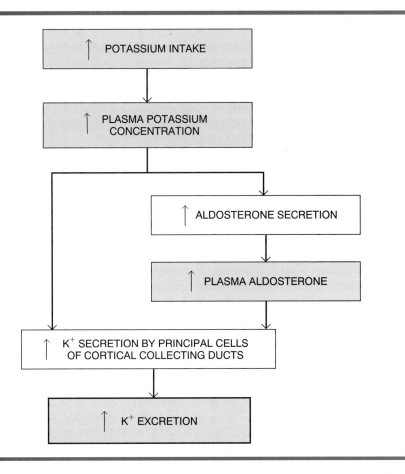

Fig. 8-2 Pathways by which an increased potassium intake induces increased potassium excretion by increasing the potassium secretion by principal cells in the cortical collecting duct.

in the principal cells; this reduces potassium secretion and excretion, thereby helping to reestablish potassium balance.

A second important factor linking potassium secretion to potassium balance is the hormone **aldosterone**, which, besides stimulating tubular sodium reabsorption by the principal cells, simultaneously enhances tubular potassium secretion by these cells. The reflex by which changes in plasma volume control aldosterone production is completely different from the reflex initiated by an excess or deficit of potassium. The former, as we saw in Chapter 7, involves the renin-angiotensin system. The latter is much simpler (Fig. 8-2): The aldosterone-secreting cells of the adrenal cortex are sensitive to the potassium concentration of the extracellular fluid bathing them. Increased intake of potassium leads to increased extracellular potassium concentration, which in turn directly stimulates aldosterone production by the adrenal cortex. The resulting increase in plasma aldosterone concentration stimulates potassium secretion by the cortical collecting duct and thereby eliminates the excess potassium from the body.

Conversely, lowered extracellular potassium concentration decreases aldosterone production and thereby reduces tubular potassium secretion; less potassium than usual is excreted in the urine, thus helping to restore the normal extracellular potassium concentration.

How does aldosterone increase potassium secretion? Recall from Chapter 7 that this hormone increases the activity and/or number of luminal-membrane sodium channels and basolateral-membrane Na,K-ATPase pumps. This latter effect increases basolateral potassium transport into the cell, hence increasing intracellular potassium concentration and the gradient for movement into the lumen. But, in addition, aldosterone increases luminal-membrane permeability to potassium by increasing the activity and/or number of potassium channels in the luminal membrane, so that the concentration gradient for diffusion is more effective in driving potassium from cell to lumen.

The examples used in this section have been concerned with changes in dietary potassium intake. However, it should be emphasized that when total-body potassium balance is perturbed by primary changes in potassium output, as for example in severe diarrhea, the same mechanisms described above operate homeostatically to control potassium secretion in the cortical collecting duct and thereby help to restore potassium balance. Thus, the potassium depletion resulting from diarrhea would tend to inhibit aldosterone secretion and, hence, potassium secretion.

The phrase "tend to inhibit" in the last sentence highlights the fact that as we have seen, potassium is not the only regulator of aldosterone secretion (Fig. 8-3). It should be evident that a conflict will arise if decreases—as in the above example—or increases in *both* potassium and plasma volume occur simultaneously, since these two changes drive aldosterone production in opposite directions. Whether aldosterone increases or decreases in such situations depends on the relative magnitudes of the opposing inputs. In general, changes in sodium balance have greater effects on aldosterone secretion than do equivalent changes in potassium balance.

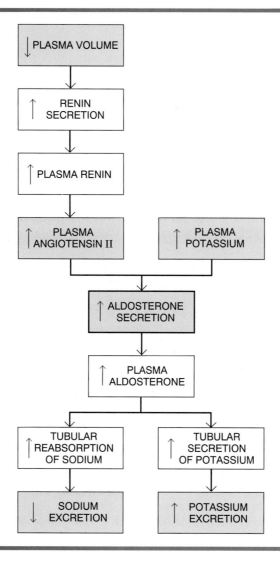

Fig. 8-3 Summary of the control of aldosterone by plasma volume and plasma potassium concentration and the effects of aldosterone on renal handling of sodium and potassium. Not shown in the figure is the fact that aldosterone exerts a third effect on the tubule: It stimulates tubular hydrogen-ion secretion, as described in Chapter 9.

This raises a potential problem for potassium homeostasis: If aldosterone secretion is altered, via the renin-angiotensin system, because of altered *sodium* balance, will the change in plasma aldosterone cause an imbalance of body *potassium* by inducing inappropriate changes in potassium secretion? In most physiological situations the answer is *no*. The explanation for this is given in the next section.[10]

Potassium Secretion and Fluid Delivery to the Cortical Collecting Duct

To answer the question raised in the previous paragraph, we must first introduce what seems like an unrelated fact: An increased delivery of fluid to the cortical collecting duct causes this tubular segment to increase its secretion of potassium. The mechanism is as follows: Recall that the final step in potassium secretion—movement across the luminal membrane—is a passive process driven by the concentration gradient for potassium from cell to lumen. A large volume of flow through the cortical collecting duct, just by its diluting effect, keeps the luminal potassium concentration low as potassium enters from the cell, and so the gradient for passive entry is maintained at a high value. Therefore, luminal entry is enhanced.

It is this relationship between fluid delivery and potassium secretion that permits changes in aldosterone caused by sodium imbalance to regulate sodium without perturbing potassium. Let us take an example (Fig. 8-4). A person on a high-sodium diet has a low plasma aldosterone concentration because of decreased renin secretion, and this will tend to decrease potassium secretion. Simultaneously, however, the person on the high-sodium diet has both increased GFR and reduced proximal sodium reabsorption (because of reductions in renal interstitial hydraulic pressure, angiotensin II, and renal sympathetic input), resulting in increased fluid delivery to the more distal tubular segments. The increased fluid flow through the cortical collecting duct tends to increase potassium secretion. The net result is that the effects on potassium secretion of the low aldosterone and high fluid delivery essentially counterbalance each other and little if any change in potassium secretion and, hence, excretion occurs. Thus, the decreased aldosterone caused by increased sodium intake can increase sodium excretion without producing significant potassium retention.

This same explanation, in reverse, applies to sodium-depleted persons and to persons with congestive heart failure or other diseases of secondary hyperaldosteronism (you might need to review, in Chapter 7, why renal function in all these categories is similar). Such persons have high aldosterone, which will tend to increase potassium secretion, but they also have low fluid delivery to the cortical collecting duct, which will tend to reduce potassium secretion. The net effect is relatively unchanged potassium secretion and excretion.[11]

To summarize, changes in aldosterone secretion—in either direction—caused by changes in sodium balance do not usually cause major perturbations in potassium balance. The reason is that these situations are usually associated with cortical-collecting-duct flows that oppose the effect of the altered aldosterone on potassium secretion.

Effects of Diuretics   We introduced the fact that increased fluid flow to the cortical collecting duct increases potassium secretion in the context of aldosterone and "conflicts" between sodium and potassium balance in order to

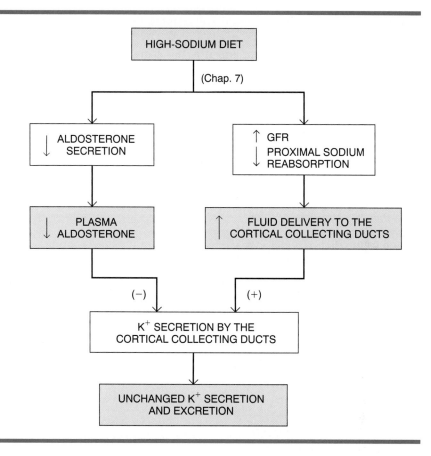

Fig. 8-4 A high-sodium diet decreases plasma aldosterone (via the renin-angiotensin system) but simultaneously increases fluid delivery to the cortical collecting duct. These inputs have opposing effects on potassium secretion by the principal cells of the cortical collecting duct, so that little change occurs.

stress the *physiological* role of the altered flow. Now, however, we must emphasize that the most striking clinical manifestation of this relationship is a pathophysiological one: Potassium excretion is almost always increased in persons undergoing osmotic diuresis or treatment with diuretics that act on the proximal tubule, loop of Henle, or distal convoluted tubule. The potassium loss may cause severe potassium depletion.

The increased potassium excretion is due partly to the fact that, as noted earlier in this chapter, potassium reabsorption in the proximal tubule and Henle's loop is linked indirectly to sodium reabsorption. Accordingly, diuretics that act on these sites inhibit not only sodium reabsorption but also potassium reabsorption. However, most of the increased potassium excretion is due not to this decreased reabsorption but to increased potassium secretion by the cortical collecting duct. In all these diuretic states, the volume of fluid flowing into the collecting duct per unit time is increased by the upstream inhibition of sodium and water reabsorption, and it is this increased flow that drives increased potassium secretion and, hence, excretion (Fig. 8-5).

To reinforce this point further, let us integrate this information with that in the previous section on aldosterone. As stated there, the elevated aldosterone in persons with heart failure or other diseases of secondary hyperaldosteronism generally does not cause potassium hypersecretion, because these people simultaneously have low fluid delivery to the cortical collecting duct. But what happens when such persons are treated with diuretics to eliminate their re-

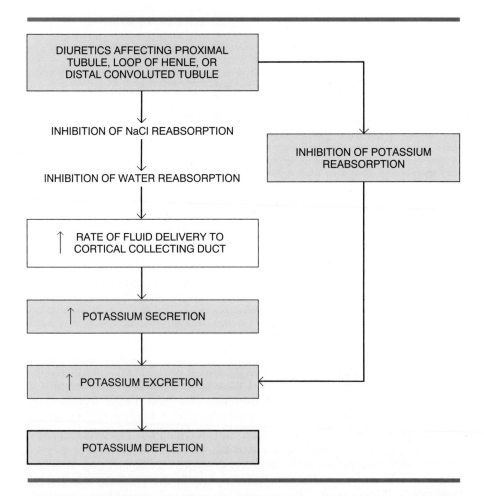

Fig. 8-5 Pathway by which diuretic drugs affecting the proximal tubule, loop of Henle, or distal convoluted tubule cause potassium depletion. The decrease in potassium reabsorption is a less important factor in causing the increased potassium excretion than the increased secretion by the principal cells of the cortical collecting ducts.

tained sodium and water? The diuretics increase fluid delivery to the cortical collecting ducts, and now the person has both increased aldosterone and increased flow to the cortical collecting duct. This combination tends to cause marked increases in potassium secretion and excretion. To prevent this combination, drugs that block the renal actions of aldosterone may be given; such drugs are diuretic because they block aldosterone's stimulation of sodium reabsorption, but, unlike other diuretics, they are "potassium-sparing" because they simultaneously block aldosterone's stimulation of potassium secretion. Another class of "potassium-sparing" diuretics blocks sodium channels in the cortical collecting duct; this prevents sodium entry from lumen to cell and effectively prevents the basolateral-membrane Na,K-ATPase pumps from transporting either sodium or potassium.

ADH and Water Diuresis Finally, it should be noted that the *water diuresis* that accompanies low plasma ADH, unlike the diuretic situations described in the previous section, is *not* associated with increased potassium secretion despite the fact that there is an increased flow through the cortical collecting duct because water reabsorption by this segment is reduced due to the low ADH. This increased flow should, therefore, cause increased secretion and excretion of potassium, but it does not. The reason stems from the fact, not given previously in the text, that ADH itself *directly stimulates* potassium secretion (by increasing the activity of luminal-membrane potassium channels). Accordingly, there are counterbalancing effects during water diuresis (Fig. 8-6): (1) Increased flow tends to cause increased potassium secretion; but (2) the absence of ADH's direct effect tends to cause decreased potassium secretion. The net result is virtually no change in potassium secretion.

Conversely, when plasma ADH is elevated there is a low flow through the cortical collecting ducts, and the effect of this low flow to reduce potassium secretion is offset by the direct stimulatory effect of ADH on potassium secretion. In essence, then, ADH is not a *primary* regulator of potassium secretion but rather prevents changes in tubular flow due to altered bodily water balance from causing potassium imbalance.

This completes the various renal effects of ADH presented in this book. They are summarized in Table 8-2.

THE EFFECTS OF ACID-BASE CHANGES ON POTASSIUM SECRETION

The previous section explained how primary changes in sodium balance usually fail to perturb potassium balance. Now we shall see that such is *not* the case for primary changes in hydrogen-ion balance. Indeed, primary acid-base disturbances are a major cause of secondary potassium imbalance because they cause marked changes in potassium secretion and excretion.

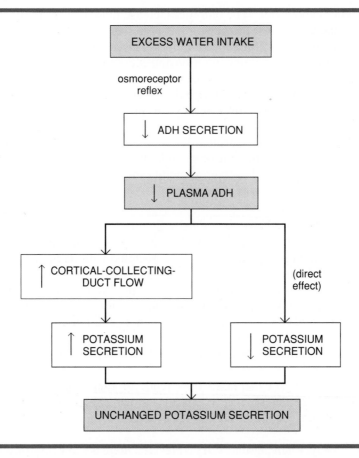

Fig. 8-6 Explanation of how water diuresis, unlike most other diureses, does *not* cause increased potassium secretion by the principal cells of the cortical collecting ducts.

Table 8-2 Summary of the Effects of ADH on Renal Function

1 Acts on principal cells of the collecting-duct system to cause:
   a Increased water reabsorption (Chapter 6)
   b Increased sodium reabsorption (synergizes with aldosterone) (Chapter 7)
   c Increased potassium secretion (Chapter 8)
2 Acts on inner medullary collecting-duct cells to cause increased urea reabsorption (Chapter 5)
3 In high concentration, constricts afferent and efferent arterioles, causing decreases in RBF and GFR, the former greater than the latter (Chapter 2)

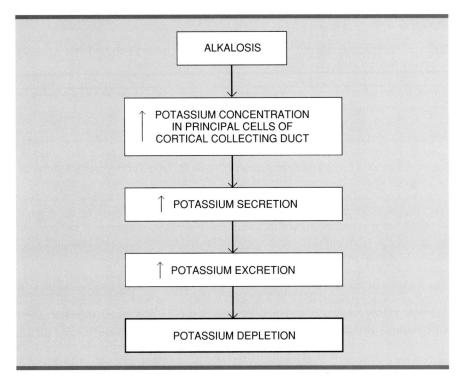

Fig. 8-7 Pathway by which alkalosis causes potassium depletion. At least one mechanism by which alkalosis increases cell concentration of potassium is stimulation of the basolateral-membrane Na,K-ATPase pumps.

The most important empirical finding is as follows: The existence of an elevated plasma pH (alkalosis) induces increased potassium secretion and excretion (Fig. 8-7).[12] Thus, a patient suffering from alkalosis (induced, say, by vomiting) will manifest increased urinary excretion of potassium solely as a result of the alkalosis and will, therefore, become potassium-deficient. How does an alkalosis stimulate potassium secretion? A major mechanism is that alkalosis stimulates the basolateral-membrane Na,K-ATPase pumps in the cortical collecting duct.[13]

What about the presence of an acidosis—does it do just the opposite, i.e., reduce potassium secretion and thereby cause potassium retention? For reasons that are still unclear no simple generalization analogous to the effect of alkalosis on potassium secretion is possible.[14]

Finally, it should be emphasized that the relationships described here are only one side of the coin. We shall describe in the next chapter how primary changes in potassium balance induce secondary changes in the renal handling of hydrogen ions.

Study questions: 57 to 60, and 62

NOTES

[1] Aldosterone was long thought to have a similar effect, but present evidence indicates that this is not the case. (See Rosa et al. in Suggested Readings.)

[2] There are many exceptions to these generalizations. (See Androgue and Madias in Suggested Readings.)

[3] For simplicity and because the process does not really alter the amount of potassium excreted, I have not described the recycling of potassium that occurs in Henle's loop. This is similar to that described for urea in Chapter 4. Potassium reabsorbed from the thick ascending limb and medullary collecting duct diffuses into the straight proximal tubule and thin limbs of Henle's loop, only to be reabsorbed once again downstream. Thus, the thick ascending limb really reabsorbs not only 30 percent of the filtered potassium but much of the potassium that is recycling. For a discussion of the possible function of this potassium recycling, see Stanton and Giebisch, and Wright and Giebisch in Suggested Readings.)

[4] The lumen-positive potential across the later proximal tubule also contributes to potassium reabsorption by diffusion. In addition, some reabsorption is caused by solvent drag. Finally, there is also some active reabsorption of potassium (the mechanism is not known). (See Stanton and Giebisch in Suggested Readings.)

[5] Some of the potassium entering across the luminal membrane by this cotransporter simply diffuses back into the lumen across luminal-membrane potassium channels rather than traversing the basolateral membrane to complete the reabsorption. For this reason, the cotransporter achieves much less reabsorption of potassium than it does of sodium and chloride.

[6] This statement is generally true for the overall contribution of the entire medullary collecting duct. However, this tubular segment, as mentioned earlier, is not a single homogenous structure, and there is considerable variability in how its different components handle potassium. (See Wright and Giebisch in Suggested Readings.)

[7] During potassium depletion there may be some regulatory stimulation of potassium reabsorption in both the cortical and medullary collecting ducts. (See Wright and Giebisch in Suggested Readings.)

[8] As noted in the legend for Fig. 8-1 there are also some luminal-membrane K,Cl cotransporters (not shown in the figure) which transport additional potassium into the lumen. This cotransporter also exists in distal convoluted tubule cells and participates, along with luminal potassium channels, in potassium secretion by this tubular segment. In addition, because it moves chloride into the lumen along with potassium, it opposes the reabsorption of chloride and can, under certain circumstances, yield net chloride secretion by these distal tubular segments. (See Wright and Giebisch in Suggested Readings.)

[9] To repeat, it is the individual *luminal-membrane* potential that opposes the luminal step in transcellular potassium secretion. In contrast, the *transtubular* potential, being lumen-negative (50 mV) in the cortical collecting duct, favors paracellular potassium

secretion by diffusion; this is probably very minor, however, because this tubular segment is "tight" and has a low ionic conductance.

[10]What about the second potential problem: When plasma aldosterone is increased because of positive potassium balance, does this cause increased sodium reabsorption and a positive bodily-sodium balance? The answer is *no*. One reason is that there are so many other controls over sodium excretion, but another is a fact not mentioned in Chapter 7: An increased plasma potassium concentration, as in positive potassium balance, inhibits proximal-tubular sodium reabsorption. Thus, this inhibition of the proximal tubule counterbalances the increased sodium reabsorption caused by aldosterone downstream in the cortical collecting duct.

[11]Contrast this result to the patient with primary hyperaldosteronism. This person has both elevated aldosterone and normal or increased delivery of fluid to the cortical collecting duct (review the changes in renal sodium handling that occur in primary hyperaldosteronism—Chapter 7) and so suffers a marked and persistent elevation in potassium secretion and excretion, enough to cause serious potassium depletion.

[12]In addition to stimulating potassium secretion alkalosis may *inhibit potassium reabsorption* by the cortical collecting duct (by inhibiting the luminal-membrane H,K-ATPase). (See Wingo and Cain in Suggested Readings.)

[13]There are probably several other mechanisms as well. Alkalosis may increase the activity and/or number of luminal-membrane potassium channels and may also enhance the cotransport of potassium and chloride from cell to lumen. (See Wright and Giebisch in Suggested Readings.)

[14]In respiratory acidosis and certain forms of metabolic acidosis (see Chapter 9 for definitions of these terms), potassium secretion is indeed decreased but only during the most acute states, usually for less then 24 h. In other forms of metabolic acidosis there may not even be an acute retention phase. But the really surprising fact is that even respiratory acidosis and those forms of metabolic acidosis that *do* manifest acute reductions in potassium secretion usually come ultimately to manifest *increased* potassium secretion, just as in alkalosis. Attempts have been made to explain these phenomena, but at the moment the mechanisms by which chronic acidosis alters renal potassium handling remain unclear. (See Wright and Giebisch in Suggested Readings.)

RENAL REGULATION OF HYDROGEN-ION BALANCE

9

Objectives

The student describes the sources of hydrogen-ion gain and loss, states the major bodily buffer systems, writes the Henderson-Hasselbalch equation for the CO_2-bicarbonate buffer system, and states in general terms the role of the kidneys in regulating extracellular pH.

The student understands the renal excretion of bicarbonate:

1 States the three renal processes that determine bicarbonate excretion

2 Calculates the mass of bicarbonate filtered each day

3 Describes the acidifying effect of renal bicarbonate loss

4 Describes the mechanism of hydrogen-ion secretion

5 Describes how hydrogen-ion secretion causes bicarbonate reabsorption; states the role of carbonic anhydrase; quantifies the relative contributions of the different tubular segments to bicarbonate reabsorption; states the collecting-duct cells that secrete hydrogen ions

6 Describes the mechanism of bicarbonate secretion and states the collecting-duct cells that perform this process

The student understands how the kidneys add new bicarbonate to the blood, i.e., excrete hydrogen ions:

1 Describes how tubular hydrogen-ion secretion can add new bicarbonate to the blood, i.e., lead to the excretion of hydrogen ion

2 States the limiting urine pH

3 States the major luminal nonbicarbonate buffer and its normal rate of excretion

4 States what determines whether a secreted hydrogen ion combines in the lumen with a filtered bicarbonate or a nonbicarbonate buffer

5 States where along the tubule most combining of secreted hydrogen ions with nonbicarbonate buffers occurs

6 Describes how proximal tubular production of NH_4^+ from glutamine, followed by excretion of the NH_4^+ in the urine, contributes to the addition of new bicarbonate to the blood

7 Defines titratable acid

8 Calculates, given data, the rate at which the kidneys contribute new bicarbonate to the blood; states representative numbers for urine titratable acid, NH_4^+, and bicarbonate in normal, acidotic, and alkalotic states

Student understands the homeostatic control of renal acid-base compensation:

1 States the control of renal glutamine metabolism and NH_4^+ excretion

2 States the control of tubular hydrogen-ion secretion by P_{CO_2} and extracellular pH

3 States the effect of alkalosis on bicarbonate secretion

4 Lists the changes (increase or decrease) of hydrogen-ion secretion, titratable acid excretion, bicarbonate excretion, NH_4^+ excretion, renal addition of new bicarbonate to the blood, and plasma bicarbonate in metabolic acidosis, metabolic alkalosis, respiratory acidosis, and respiratory alkalosis

The student understands how various factors can cause the kidneys to generate or maintain a metabolic alkalosis:

1 Describes the action of aldosterone, extracellular-volume contraction, and chloride depletion on bicarbonate reabsorption and the capacity of the kidneys to repair an alkalosis

2 States the effect of increased aldosterone alone on hydrogen-ion secretion

3 States the effect of potassium depletion alone on hydrogen-ion secretion

4 Describes how a combination of aldosterone excess and potassium depletion generates a metabolic alkalosis

5 States four factors that could contribute to a metabolic alkalosis in a person receiving diuretic drugs

The regulation of total-body hydrogen-ion balance can be viewed in the same way as the balance of any other ion—as the matching of gains and losses (Table 9-1). Not shown in the table is the gastrointestinal absorption of ingested acids or bases, which is usually a negligible factor (except in individuals who deliberately ingest large quantities of bicarbonate or some other acid or base).

Normally, the major route for gain is the generation of hydrogen ions within the body. A huge quantity of CO_2 (15,000 to 20,000 mmol) is generated

Table 9-1   Sources of Hydrogen-Ion Gain and Loss

Gain
1   Generation of hydrogen ions from CO_2 in tissue capillaries
2   Production of nonvolatile acids from the metabolism of protein and other organic molecules
3   Gain of hydrogen ions because of loss of bicarbonate in diarrhea or other nongastric gastrointestinal fluids
4   Gain of hydrogen ions because of loss of bicarbonate in urine

Loss
1   Recombination of hydrogen ions and bicarbonate in pulmonary capillaries
2   Utilization of hydrogen ions in the metabolism of organic anions
3   Loss of hydrogen ions in vomitus
4   Loss of hydrogen ions in urine

daily as the result of oxidative metabolism and yields hydrogen ions via the following reactions:

$$CO_2 + H_2O \rightleftharpoons H_2CO_3 \rightleftharpoons HCO_3^- + H^+ \qquad (9\text{-}1)$$

But this source does not normally constitute a net gain of hydrogen ions since all those hydrogen ions generated via these reactions during passage of blood through the tissues are reincorporated into water when the reactions are reversed during passage of blood through the lungs. Net retention of CO_2, however, as in hypoventilation, does result in a net gain of hydrogen ions. Conversely, net loss of CO_2, as in hyperventilation, causes net elimination of hydrogen ions.

The body also produces acids, both organic and inorganic, from sources other than CO_2. These are termed **nonvolatile acids** or **fixed acids**, to distinguish them from those produced from CO_2. These acids include: sulfuric acid and phosphoric acid, generated during the catabolism of proteins and other organic molecules containing sulfur and phosphorus; and organic acids, such as lactic acid, ketone bodies, and others. Dissociation of all these acids yields anions and hydrogen ions. But simultaneously, the metabolism of a variety of organic anions *utilizes* hydrogen ions and produces bicarbonate.[1] Thus, metabolism of "nonvolatile" solutes both generates and utilizes hydrogen ions. In the United States, where the diet is high in protein, the generation of nonvolatile acids usually predominates, and there is a net daily production in most people of 40 to 80 mmol of hydrogen ions. In contrast, in people whose diet is mainly vegetarian, metabolic utilization of hydrogen ions, with production of an equivalent amount of bicarbonate, predominates, i.e., the nonvolatile metabolic contribution is one of net loss of hydrogen ions.

A third potential source of net bodily gain or loss of hydrogen ions is the gastrointestinal secretions leaving the body. Vomitus contains a high concentration of hydrogen ions and so constitutes a source of net loss. In contrast, the other gastrointestinal secretions are alkaline and contain a higher concentration of bicarbonate than exists in plasma. Loss of these fluids, as in diarrhea, in essence constitutes a bodily gain of hydrogen ions. This is a very important point: Given the reversible equations shown in Eq. 9-1, the *loss* of a bicarbonate ion from the body has virtually the same net result as *gaining* a hydrogen ion, because loss of the bicarbonate causes the reactions to be driven to the right, thereby generating a hydrogen ion. Similarly, the *gain* of a bicarbonate by the body has virtually the same net result as *losing* a hydrogen ion, since the reaction will be driven to the left.

The urine constitutes the fourth source of net hydrogen-ion gain or loss. As is the case for the other inorganic ions described in this book, the renal excretion of hydrogen ions is regulated to achieve a stable balance and, hence, maintain a relatively stable hydrogen-ion concentration of the extracellular fluid. Thus, the kidneys normally excrete the 40 to 80 mmol of hydrogen ion generated by the average American diet. In contrast, they excrete the required amount of bicarbonate in a person whose metabolism is generating net alkali rather than net hydrogen ion. The kidneys also *adjust* their excretion of hydrogen ion and bicarbonate to compensate for any net retention or elimination of CO_2, for any increase in the metabolic production of hydrogen ions (as in diabetic ketoacidosis, for example), and for any increased loss of hydrogen ion or bicarbonate via the gastrointestinal tract. However, it should be recognized that the kidneys, instead of homeostatically regulating extracellular hydrogen-ion concentration, can themselves create an abnormal hydrogen-ion concentration by excreting too little or too much hydrogen ion.

The idea that hydrogen-ion regulation involves the same kind of input-output balancing as does that of sodium and other ions is easily obscured by the phenomenon of buffering. Between their generation and their elimination, most hydrogen ions are buffered by extracellular and intracellular buffers, i.e., they seem to disappear in a way that sodium ions do not. The normal extracellular fluid pH of 7.4 corresponds to an actual hydrogen-ion concentration of only 40 nmol/L. Without buffering interposed between generation and excretion, the daily net production rate (40–80 mmol) of only the nonvolatile acids— amounting to millions of nanomoles (1 millimole = 1 million nanomoles)— would cause huge changes in pH. Buffering minimizes these changes in hydrogen-ion concentration. But buffering does not actually eliminate the hydrogen ions from the body or retain them. This is the function of the kidneys.

The only important *extracellular* buffer is the CO_2-HCO_3^- system. The major *intracellular* buffers are phosphates and proteins, including hemoglobin. Because all these buffer systems are in equilibrium with one another, a change in one buffer pair will be associated with changes in the others. Accordingly, even though the intracellular buffers account for 50 to 90 percent of the buffering of excess hydrogen ions (depending on the source of the hydrogen ions), the emphasis in describing the overall regulation of the pH of the bodily fluids is, for a variety of reasons, generally on the CO_2-HCO_3^- system. The major reason is that there are extremely precise physiological mechanisms for regulating the two critical components of the CO_2-HCO_3^- system; the P_{CO_2} is regulated by the respiratory system, and the plasma bicarbonate concentration by the kidneys. As should be evident from the Henderson-Hasselbalch form of the equation, regulation of the P_{CO_2} and bicarbonate concentration achieves regulation of the pH:

$$pH = 6.1 + \log\left(\frac{HCO_3^-}{0.03\,P_{CO_2}}\right)$$

(The 0.03 in the equation is simply to convert the CO_2 units from mmHg to mmol/L.)

To reiterate, the kidneys contribute to the homeostasis of extracellular fluid hydrogen-ion concentration by regulating plasma bicarbonate concentration. They do so in two ways: (1) excretion of filtered and/or secreted bicarbonate, and (2) addition of *new* bicarbonate to the blood flowing through the kidneys. The kidneys can lower plasma bicarbonate concentration by excreting bicarbonate in the urine, or they can raise plasma bicarbonate concentration by producing new bicarbonate and adding it to the blood flowing through the kidneys.

Thus, in response to a lowering of plasma hydrogen-ion concentration (**alkalosis**), the kidneys excrete large quantities of bicarbonate in the urine, thereby raising plasma hydrogen-ion concentration (recall that the excretion of a bicarbonate in the urine has virtually the same effect on the blood as would adding a hydrogen ion to the blood).

In contrast, in response to a rise in plasma hydrogen-ion concentration (**acidosis**), the kidneys do not excrete bicarbonate in the urine but instead add new bicarbonate to the blood, thereby lowering the plasma hydrogen-ion concentration. As we shall see, the renal addition of new bicarbonate to the blood is associated with the excretion of an equal amount of hydrogen ions in the urine. "The kidney has added new bicarbonate to the blood," and "The kidney has *excreted* hydrogen ions" are synonymous statements. Thus, to compensate for acidosis, the kidneys excrete acid urine and alkalinize the blood; in response to alkalosis, they excrete bicarbonate-containing alkaline urine and acidify the blood.

Let us now look at how the kidneys perform these actions—either bicarbonate excretion or bicarbonate addition to the blood.

BICARBONATE EXCRETION

Urinary bicarbonate excretion is the result of bicarbonate filtration, reabsorption, and secretion:

Excreted HCO_3^-/day =

HCO_3^- filtered + HCO_3^- secreted − HCO_3^- reabsorbed

For the moment we shall ignore bicarbonate secretion and focus only on filtration and reabsorption.

Bicarbonate Filtration and Reabsorption

Bicarbonate is completely filterable at the renal corpuscles. How much is normally filtered per day?

$$\text{Filtered } HCO_3^-/\text{day} = GFR \times P_{HCO_3^-}$$
$$= 180 \text{ L/day} \times 24 \text{ mmol/L}$$
$$= 4320 \text{ mmol/day}$$

Excretion of this bicarbonate would be equivalent to adding more than 4 L of 1 N acid to the body! It is essential, therefore, that in individuals on an average American diet, virtually all the filtered bicarbonate be reabsorbed or else the body fluids would become profoundly acidic. Thus, the reabsorption of bicarbonate is an essential conservation process.

Bicarbonate reabsorption is an active process, but it is not accomplished in the conventional manner simply through an active transporter for bicarbonate ions at either the luminal or basolateral membrane. Rather, the mechanism by which bicarbonate is reabsorbed involves the tubular secretion of hydrogen ions. Let us look first at the basic process of hydrogen-ion secretion and then apply it to bicarbonate reabsorption.

Hydrogen-ion secretion occurs mainly in the proximal tubule, thick ascending limb of Henle's loop, and collecting-duct system. In contrast to the situation for sodium, water, and potassium, the collecting-duct cells that secrete hydrogen ion are the type-A intercalated cells, not the principal cells.

The basic pattern followed in all these tubular segments is the same (although the precise transporters involved differ to some extent) and is illustrated in Fig. 9-1A. Within the cells a hydrogen ion and a hydroxyl ion are generated from water. The hydrogen ion is actively secreted into the tubular lumen; the hydroxyl ion left behind inside the cell combines with CO_2 to form a bicarbonate, in a reaction catalyzed by **carbonic anhydrase**. The bicarbonate moves "downhill" across the basolateral membrane into the interstitial fluid and then into the peritubular-capillary blood. The net result is that, for every hydrogen ion secreted into the lumen, a bicarbonate enters the blood in the peritubular capillaries.

Although the pathway illustrated in Fig. 9-1A is biochemically the most likely one followed, in subsequent figures we shall use the more traditional pathway shown in Fig. 9-1B. In this schema, the hydrogen ion to be secreted is generated from H_2CO_3, and the role of carbonic anhydrase is to catalyze the formation of H_2CO_3 from H_2O and CO_2. We have chosen this schema because it is easier to visualize and it retains a role for carbonic anhydrase more familiar to the student.

Specific transporters are required for the transmembrane movements of both the hydrogen ion and the bicarbonate. Active transport of hydrogen ion across the luminal membrane from cell to lumen is achieved by three distinct luminal-membrane transporters: (1) A primary active H-ATPase exists in all the hydrogen-ion secreting tubular segments. (2) In addition, the proximal

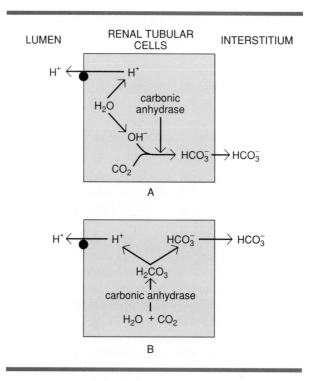

LUMEN   RENAL TUBULAR   INTERSTITIUM
                    CELLS

A

B

Fig. 9-1   Two views of tubular hydrogen-ion secretion. In both (1) a hydrogen ion is formed in the cell and actively secreted into the lumen; (2) a bicarbonate ion is formed in the cell and leaves the cell passively to enter the interstitial fluid and, from there, the peritubular-capillary blood; (3) carbonic anhydrase catalyzes the essential reaction. For simplicity in this generalized figure (and several subsequent ones), only one of the types of hydrogen-ion transporters—the H-ATPase—is shown, and the mechanism of passive bicarbonate transport across the basolateral membrane is not specified (see text, Fig. 6-1, and Fig. 9-2).

tubule and thick ascending limb of Henle's loop possess large numbers of Na/H countertransporters, as described in Chapter 6 (see Fig. 6-1); thus, most of the hydrogen-ion secretion by these segments is secondary active, driven by sodium reabsorption. (3) The type-A intercalated cells of the collecting-duct system, in addition to their primary active H-ATPase, possess a primary active H,K-ATPase, which simultaneously moves hydrogen ions into the lumen and potassium into the cell, both actively (Fig. 9-2).[2] Note that, as described in Chapter 8, the luminal-membrane H,K-ATPase also mediates active potassium reabsorption by these cells.

The basolateral-membrane "downhill" exit step for bicarbonate is via Cl/HCO$_3$ countertransporters (Fig. 9-2) or Na/HCO$_3$ cotransporters (Fig. 6-1),[3] depending on the tubular segment.

Figure 9-3 illustrates how the process of hydrogen-ion secretion shown in Fig. 9-1 achieves bicarbonate reabsorption. Once in the tubular lumen, a se-

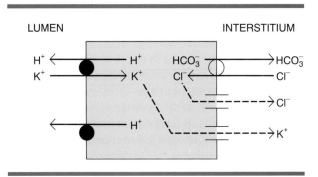

Fig. 9-2 Model of hydrogen-ion secretion by type-A intercalated cells of the collecting-duct system. This cell type possesses both H-ATPases and H,K-ATPases in its luminal membranes. Bicarbonate exits the cell "downhill" via Cl/HCO_3 countertransporters (which are identical to the band-3 erythrocyte countertransporter). Note that in addition to secreting hydrogen ions this cell actively reabsorbs potassium, as stated in Chapter 8.

creted hydrogen ion combines with a *filtered bicarbonate* to form carbonic acid. This breaks down to water and carbon dioxide, which diffuse into the cell (and can be used by the cell in another cycle). The overall result is that the bicarbonate filtered from the blood at the renal corpuscle has disappeared, but its place in the blood has been taken by the bicarbonate that was produced inside

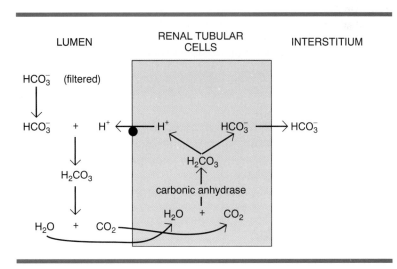

Fig. 9-3 General mechanism by which filtered bicarbonate is reabsorbed. In studying this figure, begin with the carbon dioxide and water in the tubular cells. Not shown in this generalized figure is the fact that in the proximal tubule, but not elsewhere, the breakdown of H_2CO_3 to CO_2 and H_2O *in the lumen* is catalyzed by carbonic anhydrase present in the luminal membrane.

the cell, and so no net change in plasma bicarbonate concentration has occurred. It may seem inaccurate to refer to this process as bicarbonate "reabsorption" since the bicarbonate that appears in the peritubular capillary is not the same bicarbonate that was filtered. Yet the overall result is, in effect, the same as it would be if the filtered bicarbonate had been more conventionally reabsorbed, like a sodium or potassium ion.

It is also important to note that the hydrogen ion that was *secreted* into the lumen is *not excreted* in the urine. It has been incorporated into water. The key point here is that any secreted hydrogen ion that combines with bicarbonate in the lumen to cause bicarbonate reabsorption does not contribute to the urinary excretion of hydrogen ions.

Through its secretion of hydrogen ions the proximal tubule reabsorbs approximately 80 percent of the filtered bicarbonate. The thick ascending limb of Henle's loop reabsorbs another 10 to 15 percent, and almost all the remaining bicarbonate is normally reabsorbed by the distal convoluted tubule and collecting-duct system.

Throughout the tubule, as shown in Fig. 9-1, *intracellular* carbonic anhydrase is involved in the reactions generating hydrogen ion and bicarbonate. In the proximal tubule, carbonic anhydrase is *also* located in the luminal cell membranes, and this carbonic anhydrase catalyzes the *intraluminal* decomposition of the very large quantities of carbonic acid formed in this tubular segment.[4]

Another important point needs to be made about bicarbonate reabsorption by the proximal tubule: There exists excellent glomerulotubular balance for bicarbonate reabsorption analogous to that described in Chapter 7 for sodium. When there is an increased filtered load of bicarbonate, whether caused by an increased GFR or an increased plasma bicarbonate concentration, the proximal tubule automatically reabsorbs approximately 80 percent. Thus there must be a built-in mechanism for increasing proximal-tubular hydrogen-ion secretion when filtered load of bicarbonate increases.[5] As is true for sodium glomerulotubular balance, this does not mean that proximal hydrogen-ion secretion always remains exactly proportional to filtered bicarbonate load; various inputs to be described below can alter this relationship. What it *does* mean is that changes in filtered load of bicarbonate, other factors remaining unchanged, will have little effect on bicarbonate excretion. It is for this reason that we can concentrate on changes in bicarbonate reabsorption (and secretion) when analyzing the *control* of bicarbonate excretion in later sections of this chapter.

Bicarbonate Secretion

As described above, the type-A intercalated cells of the collecting-duct system reabsorb bicarbonate. In contrast, the type-B intercalated cells, which are found only in the cortical collecting duct, *secrete* bicarbonate.[6] In essence the type-B intercalated cell is a "flipped-around" type-A intercalated cell (Fig. 9-4): The H-ATPase pump is located on the *basolateral membrane*, whereas the Cl/HCO$_3$ countertransporter is on the *luminal membrane*. Accordingly,

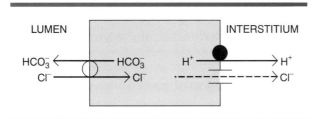

Fig. 9-4 Model of bicarbonate secretion by type-B intercalated cells. Compare this figure to Fig. 9-2, and you will see that the type-B cell is basically a "flipped-around" type-A cell. (It probably also has the expected H,K-ATPases on the basolateral membrane.) Also note that the luminal-membrane Cl/HCO$_3$ countertransporter provides the secondary active step (driven by the downhill movement of bicarbonate) for the active reabsorption of chloride by these cells, as described in Chapter 6.

bicarbonate moves "downhill" into the tubular lumen, whereas hydrogen ion is actively transported out of the cell and enters the blood, where it can combine with a bicarbonate ion. Thus, the overall process achieves disappearance of a plasma bicarbonate and excretion of a bicarbonate in the urine, with resulting acidification of the plasma and alkalinization of the urine.

For several reasons we will generally ignore bicarbonate secretion in the rest of this chapter and will refer, for the sake of simplicity, only to reabsorption, always using this term to denote *net reabsorption*—the result of bicarbonate reabsorption and secretion. First, the net handling of bicarbonate for the *entire* tubule is always profound reabsorption, never secretion. Second, experimental data are usually not available to quantify the contribution of the two unidirectional movements to observed changes in net reabsorption. Third, there are very few type-B intercalated cells in the human cortical collecting duct compared to most animal species studied, and so the importance of bicarbonate secretion may be minimal.

This completes our survey of bicarbonate excretion. Now we turn to the second way in which the kidneys can regulate plasma bicarbonate, namely, the contribution of new bicarbonate to the blood.

ADDITION OF NEW BICARBONATE TO THE BLOOD (RENAL EXCRETION OF HYDROGEN IONS)

Besides being able to conserve all the filtered bicarbonate, the kidneys can also contribute *new* bicarbonate to the blood, so that the mass of bicarbonate leaving the kidneys via the renal veins exceeds that entering the kidneys via the renal arteries. The effect of adding new bicarbonate to the body is, of course, to alkalinize it, and this is the renal compensation for acidosis.

There are two mechanisms by which the kidneys add new bicarbonate to the body: (1) secretion of hydrogen ions that, instead of causing bicarbonate reabsorption, are excreted in the urine, combined with nonbicarbonate buffers supplied by filtration; (2) catabolism of glutamine to yield ammonium (NH_4^+), followed by excretion of the NH_4^+ in the urine. We shall now describe these two mechanisms.

Hydrogen-Ion Secretion and Excretion on Urinary Buffers

We have seen how hydrogen-ion secretion achieves bicarbonate reabsorption and how this process prevents loss of filtered bicarbonate but adds no new bicarbonate to the blood. Now we shall see that the identical process of hydrogen-ion secretion can also achieve hydrogen-ion excretion and addition of new bicarbonate to the blood. Which result—whether bicarbonate reabsorption or contribution of new bicarbonate to the blood—is achieved by the secreted hydrogen ion is determined solely by the fate of this ion within the tubular lumen.

In the case of bicarbonate reabsorption, as we have seen, the secreted hydrogen ion combines with filtered bicarbonate and is incorporated into water. In contrast, in the case of the addition of new bicarbonate to the blood, the secreted hydrogen ion combines with nonbicarbonate buffers in the lumen (or to an extremely small degree, remains free in solution) and is excreted. Normally, the most important of these filtered buffers is phosphate, more specifically HPO_4^{2-}.

Figure 9-5 illustrates the sequence of events that achieves hydrogen-ion excretion on phosphate and the addition of new bicarbonate to the blood. The

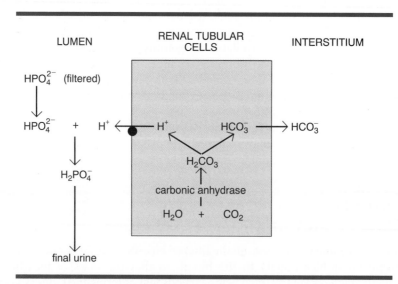

Fig. 9-5 Reaction of secreted hydrogen ion with filtered phosphate. Note that the new bicarbonate ion entering the the blood is a net gain. In contrast, Fig. 9-3 shows that no net gain of blood bicarbonate occurs when the secreted hydrogen ion is used for bicarbonate reabsorption.

process of hydrogen-ion secretion in this sequence is exactly the same as that described previously (Fig. 9-1), but the net overall effect is different simply because the secreted hydrogen ion reacts in the lumen with filtered phosphate rather than with filtered bicarbonate. Therefore, the bicarbonate generated within the tubular cell and entering the plasma constitutes a *net gain* of bicarbonate by the blood, not merely a replacement for a filtered bicarbonate. Thus, when a secreted hydrogen ion combines in the lumen with a filtered buffer other than bicarbonate, the overall effect is not merely bicarbonate conservation but rather addition to the blood of a new bicarbonate, which raises the bicarbonate concentration of the blood and alkalinizes it.

Figure 9-5 also demonstrates another important point, namely, that the renal contribution of new bicarbonate to the blood is accompanied by the *excretion* of an equivalent amount of buffered hydrogen ion in the urine. In this case, in contrast to the reabsorption of bicarbonate, the *secreted* hydrogen ion remains in the tubular fluid, trapped there by the buffer, and is *excreted* in the urine. This should reinforce the concept that when the kidneys add new bicarbonate to the blood, they are really excreting hydrogen ion from the body, thereby alkalinizing it. It must be emphasized at this point that glomerular filtration of hydrogen ions makes no significant contribution to hydrogen-ion excretion because the concentration of free hydrogen ion at a pH of 7.4, the pH of the glomerular filtrate, is less than 10^{-7}M. Even multiplying this figure by 180 L/day, one comes up with less than 0.1 mmol filtered per day.

To understand the potential contribution of various filtered buffers, as described next, it is necessary to recognize that there is a minimum urinary pH— approximately 4.4—that can be achieved. (The main reason is that the hydrogen-ion transporters are inhibited at this low pH.[7])

Phosphate and Organic Acids as Buffers To repeat, filtered phosphate is normally the most important nonbicarbonate urinary buffer. The relationship between monobasic and dibasic phosphate is as follows:

$$HPO_4^{2-} + H^+ \rightleftharpoons H_2PO_4^-$$

This buffer pair provides an excellent buffer system for urine because its pK is 6.8. Expressed in Henderson-Hasselbalch terms:

$$pH = 6.8 + \log HPO_4^{2-}/H_2PO_4^-$$

At the normal pH of plasma and, therefore, of the glomerular filtrate, the equation becomes:

$$7.4 = 6.8 + \log HPO_4^{2-}/H_2PO_4^-$$

Solving the equation, we find that there is four times more dibasic (HPO_4^{2-}) than monobasic ($H_2PO_4^-$) phosphate in plasma, and this HPO_4^{2-} is available for buffering secreted hydrogen ions. By the time the minimum intratubular pH of 4.4 is reached, virtually all the HPO_4^{2-} has been converted to $H_2PO_4^-$.

How much HPO_4^{2-} is normally filtered per day?[8]

$$\text{Total phosphate filtered/day} = 180 \text{ L/day} \times 1 \text{ mmol/L}$$
$$= 180 \text{ mmol/day}$$
$$\text{Filtered } HPO_4^{2-} = 80\% \times 180 \text{ mmol/day}$$
$$= 144 \text{ mmol/day}$$

Not all this filtered HPO_4^{2-} is available for buffering, however, because about 75 percent of filtered phosphate is reabsorbed. Accordingly, unreabsorbed HPO_4^{2-} available for buffering is 0.25×144 mmol/day $= 36$ mmol/day. Thus, the reabsorption of phosphate considerably limits the supply of HPO_4^{2-} remaining in the tubule and available for buffering.[9] Therefore, in the renal compensation for acidosis, the second mechanism for renal production of new bicarbonate—glutamine metabolism—usually bears most of the compensatory burden.

Under certain conditions various organic buffers may appear in the tubular fluid in large enough quantities to allow them also to act as important buffers. A particularly important example is the patient with uncontrolled diabetes mellitus. As a result of insulin deficiency, such a patient may become extremely acidotic because he or she produces large quantities of acetoacetic acid and β-hydroxybutyric acid, which at plasma pH almost completely dissociate to yield anions (β-hydroxybutyrate and acetoacetate) and hydrogen ions. These anions are filtered at the renal corpuscle but are only partly reabsorbed because they are present in great enough quantities to exceed the renal reabsorptive T_ms for them. Accordingly, they are available in the tubular fluid to buffer a portion of the hydrogen ions being secreted by the tubules. However, their usefulness in this role is limited by the fact that their pKs are low—approximately 4.5. This means that only about half of these anions will be titrated by secreted hydrogen ions before the limiting urine pH of 4.4 is reached, i.e., only half of them can actually be used as buffers.

Qualitative Integration of Bicarbonate Reabsorption and Hydrogen-Ion Excretion on Nonbicarbonate Buffers To repeat, a hydrogen ion secreted by the tubule can suffer one of two general fates: (1) It can combine with filtered bicarbonate, in which case the overall process accomplishes bicarbonate reabsorption (Fig. 9-3); or (2) it can combine with filtered nonbicarbonate buffers such as phosphate (Fig. 9-5). The first case is a conservation process, by which the kidneys prevent loss of bicarbonate from the body. This process alone does not alkalinize the body but rather prevents the development of an acidosis caused by bicarbonate loss. In contrast, the second process contributes new bicarbonate to the body and simultaneously excretes hydrogen ions, thereby alkalinizing the body.

What determines whether the secreted hydrogen ions, once in the lumen, combine with bicarbonate, on the one hand, or with phosphate and organic buffers, on the other? This depends on the pKs of each buffer-pair reaction and on the concentrations of each buffer present. *To simplify matters, one may assume that, compared to bicarbonate, relatively little nonbicarbonate buffer is titrated, i.e., combines with hydrogen ion, until most of the bicarbonate has been reabsorbed.* This is true mainly because the concentration of bicarbonate in the glomerular filtrate is so much higher than the concentrations of the other buffers. Once most of the filtered bicarbonate has been reabsorbed, the secreted hydrogen ions combine with the other buffers.

This analysis also explains the contributions of the different tubular segments to these processes (Table 9-2). The proximal tubule secretes very large numbers of hydrogen ions and almost all of these go to achieve bicarbonate reabsorption; as stated earlier, 80 percent of filtered bicarbonate is reabsorbed proximally. Because most of the secreted hydrogen ions are used for bicarbonate reabsorption, the pH of the luminal fluid falls less than 1 pH unit, and only a small amount of hydrogen ion is picked up by phosphate and organic buffers.

Similarly, most of the hydrogen ions secreted by the thick ascending limb of Henle's loop also go to reabsorb bicarbonate. In contrast, because so little of the filtered bicarbonate (5 to 10 percent) normally remains by the beginning of the distal convoluted tubule, the hydrogen ions secreted by this segment and the collecting-duct system can reabsorb this bicarbonate and then create the low pH required for titration of nonbicarbonate urinary buffers. However, should a large amount of bicarbonate escape proximal and loop reabsorption, most of the hydrogen ions secreted by these more distal segments, too, would be expended in reabsorbing bicarbonate rather than in titrating urinary buffers.

The fact that a marked lowering of pH and essentially complete removal of bicarbonate from the lumen occur only in the distal portions of the tubule is in keeping with another characteristic of these segments: Because they are "tight" epithelia there is little paracellular leakage of hydrogen ions from the

Table 9-2 Normal Contributions of Tubular Segments to Renal Hydrogen-Ion Balance

Proximal tubule
Reabsorbs most filtered bicarbonate (normally about 80 percent)*
Produces and secretes ammonium

Thick ascending limb of Henle's loop
Reabsorbs second largest fraction of filtered bicarbonate (normally about 10 to 15 percent)*

Distal convoluted tubule and collecting-duct system
Reabsorbs virtually all remaining filtered bicarbonate as well as any secreted bicarbonate (type-A intercalated cells)*
Produces titratable acid (type-A intercalated cells)*
Secretes bicarbonate (type-B intercalated cells)

*Denotes process achieved by hydrogen-ion secretion

lumen to the interstitium or of bicarbonate from interstitium to lumen despite very large concentration gradients favoring such leakages. For example, at a luminal pH of 4.4 there is a 1000-fold concentration difference for hydrogen ion between the renal interstitial fluid and the tubular lumen.

Glutamine Catabolism and NH_4^+ Excretion

The cells of the proximal tubule (and, to a much lesser extent, of other tubular segments) extract glutamine from both the glomerular filtrate and peritubular-capillary blood and hydrolyze it to glutamate ion and NH_4^+. Most of the glutamate is then metabolized to α-ketoglutarate, with the liberation of another NH_4^+. The subsequent metabolism of the α-ketoglutarate, either to glucose or to CO_2 and water, yields two bicarbonates. Thus, the overall yield of NH_4^+ and bicarbonate from glutamine can be written,

$$1 \text{ glutamine} \rightarrow 2 \text{ NH}_4^+ + 2 \text{ HCO}_3^-$$

The NH_4^+ is actively secreted into the lumen and excreted, whereas the bicarbonate moves into the peritubular capillaries and constitutes *new* bicarbonate (Fig. 9-6).

It is absolutely essential for the NH_4^+ produced from glutamine to be ex-creted rather than to enter the blood for the bicarbonate released into the blood truly to constitute a net gain of bicarbonate to the body. Were the NH_4^+ to enter the blood along with the bicarbonate, the two substances would rapidly be incorporated into urea or glutamine in the liver, with the disappearance of the bicarbonate from the blood.[10]

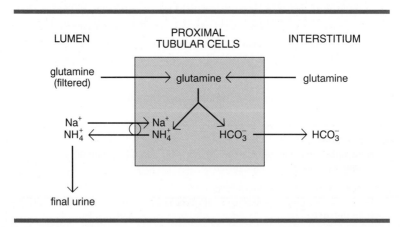

Fig. 9-6 Ammonium production and secretion by proximal tubular cells. Glutamine is transported (the mechanism is unspecified in this generalized figure) into the cells across both the luminal and basolateral membranes and is metabolized, yielding ammonium and bicarbonate. The ammonium is actively secreted into the lumen (via a Na,NH_4^+ countertransporter) and the bicarbonate moves "downhill" across the basolateral membrane.

A comparison of Figs. 9-5 and 9-6 demonstrates that the overall result—renal contribution of a new bicarbonate to the blood—is the same regardless of whether it is achieved by H^+ secretion and excretion on buffers (Fig. 9-5) or by glutamine metabolism with NH_4^+ excretion (Fig. 9-6). It is convenient, therefore, to view the latter case as representing H^+ excretion in the form of an H^+ "bound" to NH_3, just as the former case constitutes H^+ bound to phosphate or other nonbicarbonate buffers. In this manner, we can in both cases quantitatively equate the terms "H^+ excretion" and "renal contribution of new bicarbonate."

To reiterate, the NH_4^+ formed by the proximal tubular cells must be excreted if the bicarbonate simultaneously formed and moved into the blood is to remain there and constitute new bicarbonate. In fact, most of the NH_4^+ produced is indeed secreted into the lumen (the rest enters the blood instead and so is wasted), and most of this secreted NH_4^+ is ultimately excreted. The story would be simple if this proximally secreted NH_4^+ merely flowed the length of the tubule to be excreted. In reality, however, the tubular handling of NH_4^+ beyond the proximal tubule is actually a very complex sequence of transport events.[11] The only important points for us are that most of the NH_4^+ formed by the proximal tubule does end up being excreted, and that the actual percentage excreted is under physiological control.

QUANTITATION OF RENAL ACID-BASE COMPENSATION

Now we can quantitate the kidneys' contribution to hydrogen-ion balance. Said in another way, we can calculate the kidneys' net bicarbonate addition to the body or elimination from it. This value is, to say it again, identical to the kidneys' net excretion of hydrogen ions ("acid").

Such a calculation is made by answering three questions:

1. How much bicarbonate is excreted in the urine? This represents bicarbonate *loss* from the body. It is measured simply by multiplying the urine flow rate by the urinary bicarbonate concentration.
2. How much *new* bicarbonate is contributed to the plasma by secretion of hydrogen ions that end up combining in the tubular lumen with nonbicarbonate urinary buffers? This can be measured by titrating the urine with NaOH to a pH of 7.4, the pH of the plasma from which the glomerular filtrate originated. This simply reverses the events that occurred within the tubular lumen when the tubular fluid was titrated by secreted hydrogen ions. Thus, the number of milliequivalents of sodium hydroxide required to reach pH 7.4 must equal the number of millequivalents of hydrogen ion added to the tubular fluid that combined with phosphate and organic buffers. This value is known as the **titratable acid**. It must be stressed that the titratable-acid measurement does *not* pick up hydrogen ions in NH_4^+. The reason is that the pK of the ammonia-ammonium

reaction is so high (9.2) that titration with alkali to pH 7.4 will not remove hydrogen ions from NH_4^+.

3. How much *new* bicarbonate is contributed by glutamine metabolism with NH_4^+ excretion? This can be calculated by measuring urinary NH_4^+ excretion (urine flow rate × urinary NH_4^+ concentration), since for every NH_4^+ excreted, a new bicarbonate was contributed to the blood.

Thus, the data required for a quantitative assessment of the renal contribution to acid-base regulation in any person are:

1. Titratable acid excreted
2. *plus* NH_4^+ excreted
3. *minus* HCO_3^- excreted (i.e., HCO_3^- lost from the body because of incomplete reabsorption and/or HCO_3^- secretion)

Total = net HCO_3^- gain or loss to the body (negative values equal loss, positive values equal gain)

Note that there is no term for free hydrogen ion in the urine because, even at a minimum urine pH of 4.4, the number of free hydrogen ions is trivial.

Typical urine data for the amounts of bicarbonate contributed to the blood by the kidneys in the three potential acid-base states are given in Table 9-3. Note that in response to acidosis, as emphasized previously, increased production and excretion of NH_4^+ is quantitatively much more important than increased formation of titratable acid.

It should also be emphasized that the data shown for alkalosis are typical of "pure" alkalosis, i.e., alkalosis uncomplicated by other electrolyte abnormalities. As we shall see in subsequent sections, electrolyte imbalances frequently complicate the picture in alkalosis so that the expected values are not actually seen.

HOMEOSTATIC CONTROL OF RENAL ACID-BASE COMPENSATION

The patterns given in Table 9-3 are what one would predict for renal compensation for altered hydrogen-ion balance. Now we must describe the control

Table 9-3 Renal Contribution of New Bicarbonate to the Blood in Different States

	Alkalosis	Normal State	Acidosis
Titratable acid (mmol/day)	0	20	40
plus NH_4^+ excreted (mmol/day)	0	40	160
minus HCO_3^- excreted (mmol/day)	80	1	0
Total (mmol/day)	−80	59	200
	(*lost* from body)	(*added* to body)	(*added* to body)
Urine pH	8.0	6.0	4.6

mechanisms that account for these patterns (Table 9-4). What actually causes bicarbonate excretion to be increased in response to alkalosis and zero in acidosis? What causes the excretion of titratable acid and NH_4^+ to show just the opposite pattern?

Control of Renal Glutamine Metabolism and NH_4^+ Excretion

There are several homeostatic controls over the production and tubular handling of NH_4^+. First, the renal metabolism of glutamine is subject to physiological control by extracellular pH. A decrease in extracellular pH stimulates renal glutamine oxidation by the proximal tubule whereas an increase does just the opposite.[12] Thus, an acidosis, by stimulating renal glutamine oxidation, causes the kidneys to contribute more new bicarbonate to the blood, thereby counteracting the acidosis. This pH responsiveness increases over the first few days of an acidosis and allows the glutamine-NH_4^+ mechanism for new bicarbonate generation to become the preeminent renal process for opposing the acidosis. Conversely, an alkalosis inhibits glutamine metabolism, resulting in little or no renal contribution of new bicarbonate via this route.

In addition to this control of NH_4^+ *production* by pH, one or more of the complex transport processes that lead to *excretion* of the produced NH_4^+ are also influenced adaptively by extracellular pH.[13] Thus, acidosis influences NH_4^+ transport in ways that enhance excretion, whereas alkalosis does the opposite.

In conclusion, acidosis increases renal NH_4^+ synthesis and excretion, whereas alkalosis does the opposite. This explains the spectrum of changes in NH_4^+ excretion summarized in the previous section.

Control of Tubular Hydrogen-Ion Secretion

Since tubular hydrogen-ion secretion is required for both bicarbonate reabsorption and the new bicarbonate production associated with titratable acid formation, the rate of hydrogen-ion secretion is an important variable. There are many inputs that stimulate or inhibit this rate of secretion; these include changes in the P_{CO_2}, pH, volume, and ionic composition of the plasma, as well as the renal sympathetic nerves and many hormones. The effects of these

Table 9-4 Homeostatic Control of the Processes that Determine Renal Compensations for Acid-Base Disturbances

1 Glutamine metabolism and NH_4^+ excretion are increased during acidosis and decreased during alkalosis. The signal is unknown.
2 Tubular hydrogen-ion secretion is
   a Increased by the increased blood P_{CO_2} of respiratory acidosis and decreased by the decreased P_{CO_2} of respiratory alkalosis.
   b Increased, independently of changes in P_{CO_2}, by the local effects of decreased extracellular pH on the tubules; the opposite is true for increased extracellular pH.

inputs are generally to change the activity and/or number of the membrane transporters for hydrogen ion and bicarbonate in one or more of the tubular segments that secrete hydrogen ion. For example, several inputs cause an increase in the number and/or activity of H-ATPase transporters in the luminal membrane. Given the scope of this book, we can deal only with the most important inputs, skimping on the mechanisms. The interested reader can, as always, consult the Suggested Readings for further information.

Before describing these inputs, let us review what "ought" to happen (and, indeed, does) to produce the "desired" renal compensation (look again at the three data sets in Table 9-3).

When acid-base status is normal, the tubules should secrete enough hydrogen ions to achieve complete reabsorption of all filtered bicarbonate and have enough left over to form some titratable acid, thereby contributing new bicarbonate to the blood (recall that our diet usually produces net hydrogen ions, which must be covered by the kidneys' new bicarbonate). During alkalosis, tubular secretion should be too low to achieve complete reabsorption of filtered bicarbonate so that bicarbonate can be lost in the urine; no titratable acid is formed because there are no extra secreted hydrogen ions available to combine with nonbicarbonate buffers, and so no new bicarbonate is contributed to the blood. During acidosis, tubular hydrogen-ion secretion should be high enough to reabsorb all filtered bicarbonate and have enough hydrogen ions left to form increased quantities of titratable acid, thereby contributing more new bicarbonate to the blood (recall however, that this process is limited by the availability of buffers).

What, then, are the major homeostatic inputs that influence tubular hydrogen-ion secretion? They are the the arterial P_{CO_2} and the arterial pH (Table 9-4). These inputs act *directly* on the kidneys, no nerves or hormones being involved.

An increase in arterial P_{CO_2}, as occurs during respiratory acidosis, causes an increased hydrogen-ion secretion. A decrease in arterial P_{CO_2}, as occurs during respiratory alkalosis, causes a decrease in secretion. The effects are not due to the CO_2 molecule itself but to the effects of an altered arterial P_{CO_2} on renal intracellular pH. Thus, because the tubular membranes are quite permeable to CO_2, an increased arterial P_{CO_2} causes an equivalent increase in P_{CO_2} within the tubular cells. This in turn causes, by mass action, elevated intracellular hydrogen-ion concentration, and it is this change that via a sequence of intracellular events increases the rate of hydrogen-ion secretion.[14] This probably occurs in most, if not all, the tubular segments that secrete hydrogen ions.

The second signal that influences hydrogen-ion secretion in a homeostatic manner is a change in extracellular pH unrelated to P_{CO_2}. The generalization is that a decreased extracellular pH acts directly on the tubular cells, at least in part by changing intracellular pH, to stimulate hydrogen-ion secretion. An increased extracellular pH does the opposite. As with P_{CO_2}, these effects are probably exerted on most, if not all, the tubular segments that secrete hydrogen ions.

Control of Bicarbonate Secretion

I stated earlier that I would generally ignore bicarbonate secretion, which you will recall can be carried out by the type-B intercalated cells of the collecting-duct system. Little is known about the control of this process, but one fact is worth remembering: The presence of an alkalosis definitely stimulates bicarbonate secretion; the precise signal for this is not known.

Let us now apply the material covered in this section to the specific categories of acid-base disorders.

Specific Categories of Acid-Base Disorders

Renal Compensation for Respiratory Acidosis and Alkalosis

For reference, we shall present the basic equations again. [CO_2 rather than H_2CO_3 can be used in the second equation (with an appropriate change in K) because their concentrations are always in direct proportion to one another.]

$$H_2O + CO_2 \rightleftharpoons H_2CO_3 \rightleftharpoons H^+ + HCO_3^-$$
$$H^+ = K\,(CO_2/HCO_3^-)$$

In pulmonary insufficiency or hypoventilation, carbon dioxide is retained, and the resulting increase in arterial P_{CO_2} drives, by mass action, the formation of more H^+, with a resulting **respiratory acidosis**. It should be clear from the second equation that the pH could be restored to normal if the bicarbonate could be elevated to the same degree as the P_{CO_2}.[15]

It is the kidneys' job to cause this bicarbonate increase by contributing new bicarbonate to the blood. This occurs because: (1) NH_4^+ production and excretion are increased by the acidosis; and (2) the increase in both P_{CO_2} and extracellular pH stimulates renal-tubular hydrogen-ion secretion so that all filtered bicarbonate is reabsorbed and increased amounts of secreted hydrogen ion are left over for the formation of titratable acid. The renal compensation is not usually perfect, i.e., when a new steady state is reached, the plasma bicarbonate is not elevated to quite the same degree as is the P_{CO_2}. Consequently, blood pH is not returned completely to normal.

The sequence of events in response to **respiratory alkalosis**, a rise in plasma pH due to CO_2 loss, is just the opposite. Respiratory alkalosis is the result of hyperventilation, in which the person eliminates carbon dioxide faster than it is produced, thereby lowering his or her arterial P_{CO_2} and raising pH. The decreased P_{CO_2} and increase in extracellular pH reduces tubular hydrogen-ion secretion so that bicarbonate reabsorption is not complete. In addition, bicarbonate secretion is stimulated. Bicarbonate is therefore lost from the body, and the loss results in decreased plasma bicarbonate and a return of plasma pH toward normal. There is no titratable acid in the urine (which is alkaline) and little or no NH_4^+ in the urine since the alkalosis inhibits NH_4^+ production and excretion.

Renal Compensation for Metabolic Acidosis and Alkalosis

Any acid-base disturbance not caused by a primary disturbance in P_{CO_2} is called **metabolic alkalosis** or **metabolic acidosis**.

The primary cause of metabolic acidosis is either the addition to the body (by ingestion, infusion, or production) of increased amounts of any acid other than carbonic acid or, alternatively, the loss from the body of bicarbonate (as in diarrhea). Inspection of the equations reveals that either loss of bicarbonate or addition of hydrogen ions will lower both the plasma pH and the plasma bicarbonate concentration. The kidneys' compensation is to raise the plasma bicarbonate concentration back toward normal, thereby returning pH toward normal. To do this, the kidneys must reabsorb all the filtered bicarbonate and contribute new bicarbonate through increased formation and excretion of NH_4^+ and titratable acid. This is precisely what normal kidneys do, and the urines excreted in respiratory acidosis and metabolic acidosis are indistinguishable in these respects.

The increased NH_4^+ production and excretion triggered by the acidosis are predictable from previous sections, but the total reabsorption of bicarbonate and formation of increased titratable acid require more comment since the two major signals for hydrogen-ion secretion described in the previous section—P_{CO_2} and extracelluallar pH—are in opposed directions. Specifically, the extracellular pH is down (which would stimulate hydrogen-ion secretion) but the P_{CO_2} is also decreased (which would inhibit it). The reason that the P_{CO_2} is *decreased* in metabolic acidosis is that, as the arterial pH falls as a result of whatever is causing the metabolic acidosis, pulmonary ventilation is reflexly stimulated. This is, of course, the respiratory compensation for the acidosis, and its effect is to reduce arterial P_{CO_2}. Therefore, because renal-tubular cell pH is rapidly altered by changes in P_{CO_2}, renal-tubular cell pH is likely to be *increased* in the early stages of metabolic acidosis despite a decreased extracellular pH.[16]

How then can the kidneys manage fully to perform their compensatory function with the decreased P_{CO_2} opposing increased hydrogen-ion secretion? This apparent paradox is resolved when one recalls that in metabolic acidosis the plasma bicarbonate is lower than normal. Therefore, the mass of bicarbonate filtered (GFR $\times P_{HCO_3^-}$) is reduced proportionally to the decreased plasma bicarbonate, and *less* hydrogen ion "needs" to be secreted to accomplish total reabsorption of the filtered bicarbonate. Accordingly, if the signal for hydrogen-ion secretion were unchanged or even decreased because of the low P_{CO_2}, there would still be considerable hydrogen ion available after the bicarbonate had been completely reabsorbed to form titratable acid, thereby contributing new bicarbonate to the plasma. For example, compare the data on the next page for a person with metabolic acidosis with those for a normal person.

The situation in metabolic alkalosis is just the opposite. Despite a normal or even increased signal for hydrogen-ion secretion secondary to a reflexly elevated P_{CO_2}, the load of filtered bicarbonate is so great that more bicarbonate escapes reabsorption. Also, increased bicarbonate secretion occurs in metabolic alkalosis. Overall, then, bicarbonate is lost in the urine, plasma bicarbonate is decreased, and pH decreases toward normal. The urine also

	Normal	Metabolic acidosis
1 Plasma HCO_3^-	24 mmol/L	12 mmol/L
2 GFR	180 L/day	180 L/day
Filtered HCO_3^-	4320 mmol/day	2160 mmol/day
(1 × 2)		
A Reabsorbed HCO_3^-	4315 mmol/day	2160 mmol/day
B Titratable acid	20 mmol/day	80 mmol/day
Total H^+ secreted	4335 mmol/day	2240 mmol/day
(A + B)		

contains little or no NH_4^+ because NH_4^+ production and excretion are inhibited by the alkalosis.

FACTORS CAUSING THE KIDNEYS TO GENERATE OR MAINTAIN A METABOLIC ALKALOSIS

The previous sections described the mechanisms by which NH_4^+ production and hydrogen-ion secretion are controlled to achieve acid-base *homeostasis*. We now describe how factors *not* designed to maintain a constant pH can also influence these processes. In other words, just as for potassium, hydrogen-ion balance has its own distinct homeostatic controls, but it is also at the mercy of other interacting factors. The most important of these are extracellular-volume contraction, chloride depletion, and the combination of aldosterone excess and potassium depletion. The key event in all these situations is oversecretion of hydrogen ion (and sometimes of NH_4^+ as well), producing one of two general results: (1) The kidneys may *generate* a metabolic alkalosis; or (2) the kidneys may not generate a metabolic alkalosis but may fail to compensate as usual for an existing metabolic alkalosis.

Influence of Extracellular-Volume Contraction

The presence of extracellular-volume contraction because of salt depletion interferes with the ability of the kidneys to compensate for a metabolic alkalosis. In metabolic alkalosis the plasma bicarbonate is elevated, either because of the addition of bicarbonate to the body or because of the loss of hydrogen ion from it. The normal renal compensation should be to set hydrogen-ion secretion at a level that falls short of complete bicarbonate reabsorption and thereby allows the excess bicarbonate to be excreted. But the presence of the extracellular-volume contraction not only stimulates sodium reabsorption but also stimulates hydrogen-ion secretion.

There are several mechanisms that account for this stimulation. First, not mentioned previously is the fact that aldosterone, which is increased in extracellular-volume contraction, stimulates hydrogen-ion secretion.[17] This action, which is mainly on type-A intercalated cells, is distinct from (and

Table 9-5   Summary of Aldosterone's Major Renal Actions

1	Stimulates sodium reabsorption (principal cells)
2	Stimulates potassium secretion (principal cells)
3	Stimulates hydrogen-ion secretion (type-A intercalated cells)

quantitatively much less important than) aldosterone's stimulation of sodium reabsorption and potassium secretion, which is exerted on principal cells (Table 9-5).[18] Second, other as yet unidentified factors may also play a role.[19]

Whatever the mechanism, the net result is that all the filtered bicarbonate is reabsorbed so that the already elevated plasma bicarbonate associated with the preexisting metabolic alkalosis is locked in, and the plasma pH remains unchanged. The urine, instead of being alkaline, as it should be when the kidneys are normally compensating for a metabolic alkalosis, is somewhat acid.

Influence of Chloride Depletion

We referred to extracellular-volume contraction in the previous section without distinguishing between sodium and chloride losses as the cause because loss of either of these ions will lead to extracellular-volume contraction. Now, however, we must emphasize that specific chloride depletion, in a manner independent of and in addition to extracellular-volume contraction, helps maintain metabolic alkalosis by stimulating hydrogen-ion secretion and/or inhibiting bicarbonate secretion.[20] The result is that bicarbonate excretion remains essentially zero and the metabolic alkalosis is not compensated. This phenomenon has considerable clinical importance because many situations (vomiting, for example) are associated with both metabolic alkalosis and chloride depletion, as well as extracellular-volume contraction.

Influence of Aldosterone Excess and Potassium Depletion

As noted earlier, aldosterone stimulates hydrogen-ion secretion, although the effect is relatively small. Potassium depletion, by itself, also weakly stimulates tubular hydrogen-ion secretion and NH_4^+ production.[21,22] Now we come to the critical point. The combination of potassium depletion of even moderate degree and high levels of aldosterone stimulates tubular hydrogen-ion secretion markedly (NH_4^+ production also goes up significantly). As a result, the renal tubules not only reabsorb all filtered bicarbonate but also contribute inappropriately large amounts of new bicarbonate to the body, thereby causing the development of metabolic alkalosis. Note that there may have been nothing wrong with the acid-base balance to start with: The alkalosis is actually *generated* by the kidneys themselves. Of course, if alkalosis were already present because of some other cause, this high-aldosterone/potassium-depletion com-

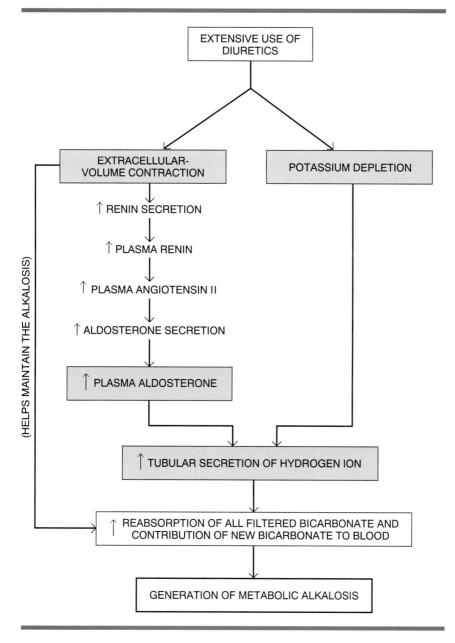

Fig. 9-7 Pathway by which overuse of diuretics leads to a metabolic alkalosis. Not shown in the figure is the fact that NH_4^+ production and excretion are also increased by the presence of a high aldosterone and potassium depletion. Note that the extracellular-volume contraction, via both aldosterone and as yet unidentified nonaldosterone mechanisms, helps to maintain the alkalosis once it has been generated. If the diuretics have also caused chloride depletion, this too will contribute to the maintenance of the metabolic alkalosis (not shown in the figure).

bination would not only prevent the kidneys from compensating but would also make the alkalosis worse.

This phenomenon is important because the combination of a markedly elevated aldosterone and potassium depletion occurs in a variety of clinical situations. One very common situation in which the two coexist is the extensive use of diuretic drugs (Fig. 9-7). This combination can then act to generate a metabolic alkalosis. Note also that the person in this example is triply in trouble: As described in the previous sections, extracellular-volume contraction per se, via multiple mechanisms, stimulates reabsorption of bicarbonate. This helps to maintain the alkalosis once the high-aldosterone/potassium-depletion combination has generated it. Indeed, if the diuretics have also produced chloride depletion in addition to the extracellular-volume contraction, the person will be quadruply in trouble because chloride depletion, as described above, causes excessive secretion of hydrogen ion.

Study questions: 61 and 63 to 68

NOTES

[1]Another large potential source of bicarbonate is protein catabolism to NH_4^+ and HCO_3^-. The NH_4^+ will not dissociate, to any significant degree, to yield hydrogen ions because the pK of the $NH_4^+ \rightleftharpoons NH_3 + H^+$ reaction is very high (9.2); accordingly, protein catabolism yields net HCO_3^-. However, virtually all the NH_4^+ and HCO_3^- formed by protein catabolism are rapidly combined to form urea in the liver, and so the HCO_3^- disappears. In other words, urea formation undoes the alkalinizing effects of protein catabolism. (We will revisit this issue, this time in the text, in the section on ammonium.) This glib explanation of how protein catabolism doesn't yield net bicarbonate is not accepted by all, however. Indeed, some have argued that the control of ureagenesis is the major regulator of acid-base balance. These scientists go so far as to argue that the kidneys play little if any role in acid-base balance (if they are right, you could simply skip the rest of this chapter). (For details on this fascinating controversy, see Walser in Suggested Readings.)

[2]The terminal portion of the inner medullary collecting duct is unusual in that it has no intercalated cells, only the cell type known as *inner medullary collecting duct cells*. The mechanism by which this segment secretes hydrogen ions is not clear.

[3]The Na/HCO_3 cotransporter is a very interesting transporter because the energy of the bicarbonate moving downhill across the basolateral membrane drives the uphill movement of sodium. Thus this is another way, besides the Na,K-ATPase, of actively transporting sodium across the basolateral membrane. Its contribution, however, is quite small, and if you trace the sequence of events back far enough (Fig. 6-1) you will see that the availability of the bicarbonates to the cotransporter is ultimately dependent on the Na,K-ATPase anyway.

[4]Although still controversial, it appears that there is little or no active luminal-membrane carbonic anhydrase in several of the segments beyond the proximal tubule. Therefore, the intraluminal breakdown of H_2CO_3 to CO_2 and H_2O occurs relatively

slowly in these segments. Therefore, much of the CO_2 formation occurs after the urine has left the tubule and entered the lower urinary tract. Here the surface-to-volume relationships are unfavorable for the diffusion of CO_2 out of the lumen. Accordingly, for this reason (and others not mentioned here), the urine P_{CO_2} can be much higher than the arterial P_{CO_2} under certain conditions. (See Dubose, Jr in Suggested Readings.)

[5]The mechanism is not fully understood. (See Hamm and Alpern in Suggested Readings.)

[6]It is likely that intercalated cells can display plasticity, i.e., that type-A and type-B cells can undergo some interconversion. The physiological importance of this possibility is not known. (See Schuster in Suggested Readings.)

[7]See Steinmetz in Suggested Readings for an explanation of this phenomenon.

[8]The number 1 mmol/L in the equation that follows is the value of phosphate in glomerular filtrate; it is somewhat lower than the plasma concentration because a small fraction of plasma phosphate is protein-bound and, therefore, not filterable.

[9]It is adaptive, therefore, that the presence of a low plasma pH (acidosis) partially inhibits phosphate reabsorption, thereby increasing the amount of luminal phosphate available for buffering. This effect is relatively modest, however. (See Hamm and Alpern in Suggested Readings for mechanisms.)

[10]Let us point out an intuitively seductive but *wrong* alternative explanation. You might think that if NH_4^+ were to enter the blood along with the bicarbonate, the NH_4^+ would directly donate a proton to the bicarbonate to yield NH_3, CO_2, and H_2O, but this cannot happen to any significant degree. Why? Because the pK of the $NH_4^+ \rightleftharpoons NH_3 + H^+$ reaction is so high (9.2), NH_4^+ donates virtually no protons at physiological pHs, i.e., NH_4^+ is not really an acid at these pHs. To emphasize these points, let us explain why the administration of NH_4Cl causes acidosis. As described in the text, the NH_4^+ that appears when the NH_4Cl dissociates does not yield H^+ and NH_3 to any significant degree. Rather, the NH_4^+ is incorporated into urea and/or glutamine, and these reactions utilize bicarbonate from the plasma. It is this disappearance of bicarbonate that causes the acidosis.

[11]These events, involving movement of both NH_3 and NH_4^+, include reabsorption from the thick ascending limb of Henle's loop into the interstitium, countercurrent multiplication of the concentrations in the medulla, and, finally, secretion into the collecting ducts and "trapping" there. (See Hamm and Alpern, and Knepper et al. in Suggested Readings.)

[12]Acidosis also causes a marked increase in hepatic glutamine synthesis, thereby supplying to the kidneys the additional glutamine required for increased renal glutamine metabolism.

[13]See Knepper et al. in Suggested Readings.

[14]At least one of the mechanisms is that the decreased intracellular pH induces the insertion of H-ATPase pumps in the luminal membrane of the cells.

[15]There is, of course, an automatic increase, by mass action, in bicarbonate concentration solely as a result of the reaction being driven to the right by the elevated P_{CO_2}, but the increase in bicarbonate concentration is not nearly as much, percentage-wise, as the rise in P_{CO_2}. If we transpose the second equation, we can see why mass action alone does not lead to proportionate increases of bicarbonate and carbon dioxide when P_{CO_2} increases:

$$(H^+) (HCO_3^-) = K(CO_2)$$

This form of the equation emphasizes that a rise in carbon dioxide causes a proportionate rise in the *product* (H^+) (HCO_3^-). Since hydrogen-ion concentration increases, bicarbonate concentration cannot increase as much as carbon dioxide does or else the (H^+) (HCO_3^-) product would rise more than proportionately. Plug in some real numbers and convince yourself that this is true.

[16] In patients with chronic metabolic acidosis, it is likely that intracellular pH returns to normal or actually decreases, despite a continued decrease in P_{CO_2}, probably because of altered basolateral-membrane transport of hydrogen ion.

[17]Aldosterone stimulates the luminal-membrane H-ATPase (and, possibly, also the H,K-ATPase). Recent evidence suggests that this hormone may also stimulate hydrogen-ion secretion by the thick ascending limb of Henle's loop. (See Hamm and Alpern in Suggested Readings.)

[18]It is likely that this action of aldosterone is part of a true homeostatic control system for regulating extracellular pH. A variety of experiments have demonstrated that acidosis, either metabolic or respiratory, stimulates renin secretion; the resulting increase in angiotensin II will stimulate aldosterone secretion, and this hormone, by its stimulation of hydrogen-ion secretion, would help eliminate the acidosis. Also, it is likely that an acidosis stimulates aldosterone secretion by a direct effect on the adrenal cortex. Finally, if you look at the next note you'll see that angiotensin II and the renal nerves, by their direct tubular effects, may further contribute to the adaptive response to acidosis independent of their role in elevating plasma aldosterone.

[19]For example, the renal nerves and angiotensin II also stimulate hydrogen-ion secretion, mainly by the proximal tubule. This effect is mediated by a stimulation of the Na/H countertransporters in this tubular segment and probably constitutes the mechanism by which the renal nerves and angiotensin II stimulate proximal sodium reabsorption, as described in Chapter 7. The Na/H countertransporter can be influenced by many hormones and paracrine agents other than angiotensin II. These include parathyroid hormone and dopamine, both of which inhibit it, and catecholamines and insulin, which stimulate it. The physiological significance of these inputs is presently unclear. (See Alpern and Rector, and Cogan and Quan in Suggested Readings.)

[20]Multiple mechanisms are probably involved in this response, which involves several tubular segments. One involves bicarbonate secretion by the type-B intercalated cells: Recall that bicarbonate secretion utilizes a Cl/bicarbonate countertransporter on the *luminal* membrane of these cells for the movement of bicarbonate from cell to lumen; this transporter is sensitive to the chloride concentration of the luminal fluid and so, during chloride depletion, is inhibited by the low luminal chloride concentra-

tion. This would cause less bicarbonate secretion and, hence, excretion than usually occurs in alkalosis.

[21]Multiple mechanisms are involved. For one thing, potassium depletion of renal-tubular cells causes a decrease in renal-cell pH (because of the reciprocal relations between cell pH and potassium described in Chapter 8), and this decrease stimulates hydrogen-ion secretion. In addition, potassium depletion stimulates the H,K-ATPase in the collecting-duct system.

[22] One reason for the failure of potassium depletion by itself to produce a large excess of hydrogen-ion secretion is that potassium depletion inhibits secretion of aldosterone (as described in Chapter 8). Accordingly, the stimulatory effect aldosterone tonically exerts on hydrogen-ion secretion is lost, and this loss offsets the stimulatory effect exerted by potassium depletion.

REGULATION OF CALCIUM AND PHOSPHATE BALANCE

10

Objectives

The student understands the regulation of calcium balance and extracellular concentration:

1 States the normal plasma calcium concentration and the percentage that is protein-bound; states the effect of pH on the free and bound fractions

2 Describes the gastrointestinal handling of calcium

3 Describes the basic renal handling of calcium; states the effects of changes in sodium intake and of acidosis on calcium excretion

4 States the percentage of total-body calcium in bone

5 Lists the effects of parathyroid hormone and their adaptive value

6 Describes the control of secretion of parathyroid hormone

7 Describes the sequence of reactions leading from 7-dehydrocholesterol to $1,25\text{-}(OH)_2D_3$; states the major control over the 1-hydroxylation step

8 Lists the effects of $1,25\text{-}(OH)_2D_3$

9 Defines calcitonin and states its suggested role in calcium regulation

10 Predicts changes in plasma and urinary calcium and phosphate in patients with hyperparathyroidism or with $1,25\text{-}(OH)_2D_3$ deficiency

The student understands the renal regulation of phosphate balance:

1 Describes the renal handling of phosphate

2 States two mechanisms that cause increased urinary phosphate excretion when dietary phosphate is elevated

3 States the effects of parathyroid hormone and $1,25\text{-}(OH)_2D_3$ on tubular reabsorption of phosphate

Extracellular calcium concentration is normally held relatively constant, the requirement for precise regulation stemming primarily from the profound effects of calcium on neuromuscular excitability. A low calcium concentration increases the excitability of nerve- and muscle-cell membranes so that individuals with low plasma calcium suffer from *hypocalcemic tetany*, characterized by skeletal muscle spasms. Hypercalcemia is dangerous too, because it causes cardiac arrhythmias as well as depressed neuromuscular excitability. All these effects reflect calcium's ability to bind to plasma-membrane proteins that function as ion channels, altering their open or closed state. This effect of calcium on membranes is totally distinct from its role as an excitation-contraction coupler.

It is important to recognize that the plasma calcium (normally 5 mEq/L or 2.5 mmol/L) exists in three general forms, in approximately the following proportions: (1) 45 percent is in the ionized (Ca^{2+}) form, the only biologically active form in nerve, muscle, and other target organs. (2) 15 percent is complexed to anions with relatively low molecular weights, such as citrate and phosphate. (3) 40 percent is reversibly bound to plasma proteins. One of the most important influences on the degree of protein binding is the plasma pH. An increase in pH causes increased calcium binding because the decreased acidity converts more of the protein to the anionic form, i.e., it exposes additional negatively charged binding sites. Thus, a patient with alkalosis is more susceptible to tetany, whereas a patient with acidosis will not manifest tetany at levels of total plasma calcium low enough to cause symptoms in normal people.

EFFECTOR SITES FOR CALCIUM HOMEOSTASIS

Normally, the body remains in stable calcium balance, i.e., the amount of ingested calcium is equal to the calcium lost in urine, feces, and sweat combined. The chapters in this book on sodium, water, potassium, and hydrogen-ion homeostasis were concerned almost entirely with the *renal* handling of these substances. In contrast, the regulation of calcium depends not only on the kidneys but also on bone and the gastrointestinal tract. We will first describe how these three effector sites handle calcium and then discuss how they are influenced by hormones in the homeostatic control of plasma calcium concentration.

Gastrointestinal Tract

In contrast to the situation for sodium, chloride, and potassium, a large fraction of ingested calcium is not normally absorbed from the intestine and simply leaves the body along with the feces. Accordingly, changes in the active transport system that moves calcium from intestinal lumen to blood can result in large increases or decreases in calcium absorption. Hormonal control of this absorptive process is the major means for homeostatically regulating total-body calcium balance.

Kidneys

The kidneys handle calcium by filtration and reabsorption. Only about 60 percent of the plasma calcium is filterable, the remainder being protein-bound. Most calcium reabsorption occurs in the proximal tubule (about 60 percent) and the remainder in the thick ascending limb of Henle's loop, distal convoluted tubule, and collecting-duct system. Overall, reabsorption is normally 97 to 99 percent.

Calcium reabsorption in the proximal tubule and thick ascending limb of Henle's loop is largely passive and paracellular, and the electrochemical forces driving it are dependent directly or indirectly on sodium reabsorption.[1] In contrast, calcium reabsorption in the more distal segments is active and transcellular (Fig. 10-1). This is where the homeostatic control of calcium reabsorption is exerted.[2]

The amount of calcium excreted is normally equal to the *net* addition of new calcium to the body via the gastrointestinal tract; thus, the kidneys help maintain a stable balance of total-body calcium. However, the kidneys respond to changes in *dietary* calcium much less than they do to changes in dietary

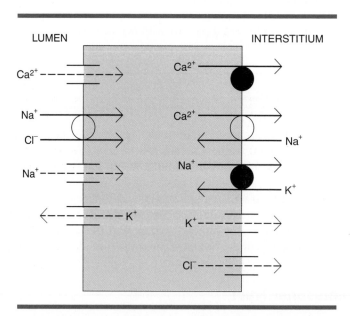

Fig. 10-1 Model of distal convoluted tubule, showing mechanisms of calcium reabsorption (as well as sodium reabsorption and potassium secretion). Calcium diffuses, via calcium channels, from the lumen into the cell down the very large electrochemical gradient that exists here, as in virtually all cells of the body. It is then actively transported out of the cell across the basolateral membrane, both by a primary active Ca-ATPase and by a Na/Ca countertransporter, the latter making use of the energy from downhill sodium movement into the cell to move calcium out.

sodium, water, or potassium. For example, only about 5 percent of an increment in dietary calcium appears in the urine. The reason is that most of the dietary increment never gains entry to the blood because it fails to be absorbed from the gastrointestinal tract. At the other end of the spectrum, when dietary intake of calcium is reduced to extremely low levels, there is a slow reduction of urinary calcium, but some continues to appear in the urine for weeks.

How do the renal homeostatic mechanisms operate? Since calcium is filtered and reabsorbed, but not secreted,

$$\text{Ca excretion} = \text{Ca filtered} - \text{Ca reabsorbed}$$

Accordingly, excretion can be altered homeostatically by changing either the filtered or the rate of reabsorption. Both occur. For example, what happens when a person increases his or her calcium intake? Transiently, intake exceeds output, positive calcium balance ensues, and plasma calcium concentration increases. This in itself increases both the filtered mass of calcium and excretion. Simultaneously, as we shall see, the increased plasma calcium triggers hormonal changes that cause a diminished reabsorption. The net result of these responses is increased calcium excretion.

A bewildering array of factors *not* designed to maintain calcium homeostasis can also influence urinary calcium excretion, mainly by stimulating or inhibiting tubular reabsorption. These include a large number of hormones, ions, acid-base disturbances, and drugs (see Suki and Rouse in Suggested Readings).

One of the most important of these influences on calcium reabsorption is sodium: An increase or decrease in urinary calcium excretion can be induced simply by administering or withholding salt, respectively. (This fact is used clinically when one wishes to decrease or increase the amount of calcium in the body). The explanation is that, as described earlier, passive calcium reabsorption in the proximal tubule and thick ascending limb of Henle's loop is dependent on sodium reabsorption.

A second very important factor that influences tubular calcium reabsorption but is not designed to maintain calcium homeostasis is the presence of an acidosis. The mechanism is not clear, but acidosis markedly inhibits calcium reabsorption and, hence, causes increased calcium excretion. Alkalosis tends to do just the opposite—enhance calcium reabsorption and reduce excretion.

Bone

The activities of the gastrointestinal tract and the kidneys determine the net intake and output of calcium for the entire body and, thereby, the overall state of calcium balance. In contrast, interchanges of calcium between extracellular fluid and bone do not alter total-body balance but, rather, the *distribution* of calcium within the body. Approximately 99 percent of the total-body calcium is contained in bone, which is basically a collagen-protein framework on which calcium phosphate (and other minerals) are deposited in a crystal structure known as **hydroxyapatite**.

Bone is not a dead, fixed tissue; rather, it is cellular and well supplied with blood. Most important, it is continuously broken down (resorbed) and simultaneously reformed under the influence of the bone cells. Normally, the rates of resorption and reformation are identical. However, we shall see that several hormones can break this balance by influencing the rates of deposition or resorption of bone calcium. Accordingly, bone provides a huge potential source or sink for the net withdrawal of calcium from or addition to extracellular fluid.

HORMONAL CONTROL OF EFFECTOR SITES

Parathyroid Hormone

The gastrointestinal tract, the kidneys, and bone are all subject to direct or indirect control by a polypeptide hormone called **parathyroid hormone**, produced by the **parathyroid glands**. The secretion of parathyroid hormone is controlled directly by the calcium concentration of the extracellular fluid bathing the cells of these glands. Decreased plasma calcium concentration stimulates parathyroid-hormone secretion, and increased plasma concentration does just the opposite. Extracellular calcium concentration acts directly on the parathyroids without any intermediary hormones or nerves.

Parathyroid hormone exerts at least four distinct effects on calcium homeostasis:

1. It increases the movement of calcium from bone into extracellular fluid by stimulating bone resorption. In this manner the immense store of calcium contained in bone is made available for the regulation of extracellular calcium concentration.
2. It stimulates the activation of vitamin D (see below), and this hormone then increases intestinal absorption of calcium.
3. It increases renal-tubular calcium reabsorption, mainly by an action on the distal convoluted tubule, and thus decreases urinary calcium excretion.[3]
4. It reduces the proximal-tubular reabsorption of phosphate, thereby raising urinary phosphate excretion and lowering extracellular phosphate concentration.

The adaptive value of the first three effects (summarized in Fig. 10-2) should be obvious: They all result in a higher extracellular calcium concentration and thus compensate for the lower calcium concentration that originally stimulated parathyroid-hormone secretion. The adaptive value of the fourth effect requires further explanation, as follows.

When parathyroid hormone induces bone resorption, both calcium and phosphate are released. Similarly, activated vitamin D enhances the intestinal

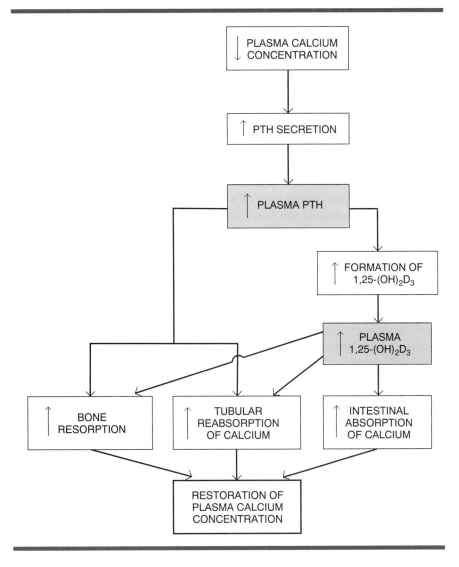

Fig. 10-2 Hormonally mediated compensatory response to reduced plasma calcium concentration. PTH = parathyroid hormone. The effects of PTH and 1,25-$(OH)_2D_3$ on phosphate are not shown in the figure (see text and Fig. 10-3).

absorption of both calcium and phosphate. Accordingly, while the low calcium, which triggered the increase in parathyroid hormone, is being homeostatically compensated, the plasma phosphate would tend to be raised above normal. However, plasma phosphate does not actually increase because of parathyroid hormone's inhibition of tubular phosphate reabsorption. Indeed, so potent is this effect that plasma phosphate may actually decrease when parathyroid-hormone levels are elevated. (This reduction in phosphate is adaptive in that it facilitates further bone resorption because of local interactions between calcium and phosphate.)

In contrast to the state described above, an increase in extracellular calcium concentration reduces parathyroid-hormone secretion and, thereby, produces increased urinary and fecal calcium loss and net movement of calcium from extracellular fluid into bone.

Parathyroid hormone has other functions in the body, but the four effects discussed above constitute the major mechanisms by which it integrates various organs and tissues in the regulation of extracellular calcium concentration.[4]

Hyperparathyroidism, resulting from a primary defect in the parathyroid glands (e.g., a hormone-secreting tumor), well illustrates the actions of parathyroid hormone. The excess hormone causes enhanced bone resorption, leading to bone thinning and the formation of completely calcium-free areas or cysts. Plasma calcium increases and plasma phosphate decreases; the latter is caused by increased urinary phosphate excretion. The increased plasma calcium is deposited in various body tissues, including the kidneys, where stones may be formed. A seeming paradox is that urinary calcium excretion is *increased* despite the fact that tubular calcium reabsorption is enhanced by parathyroid hormone. The reason is that the elevated plasma calcium concentration induced by the nonrenal effects of parathyroid hormone causes the filtered load of calcium to increase even more than does the reabsorptive rate. This result nicely illustrates the necessity of taking both filtration and reabsorption (and secretion, if relevant) into account when analyzing excretory changes of any substance.

1,25-dihydroxyvitamin D₃

The term **vitamin D** denotes a group of closely related sterols. One of these compounds, called **vitamin D$_3$** (or cholecalciferol), is formed by the action of ultraviolet radiation on 7-dehydrocholesterol in the skin. A second source of vitamin D is that ingested in food, specifically in plants. Because of clothing and decreased out-of-doors living, people are often dependent on this dietary source. The form of vitamin D found naturally in food differs only trivially in structure from vitamin D$_3$, and no distinction will be made between them in the subsequent description.

Vitamin D$_3$ is inactive and must undergo metabolic changes within the body before it can influence its target cells. It enters the blood and is hydroxylated in the 25 position by the liver and then in the 1 position by the kidneys (specifically by proximal tubular cells). The end result is the active form of vitamin D—**1,25-dihydroxyvitamin D$_3$**, abbreviated **1,25-(OH)$_2$D$_3$**. From this description, it should be evident that 1,25-(OH)$_2$D$_3$ is actually a hormone, not a vitamin, since it is made in the body.

The major action of 1,25-(OH)$_2$D$_3$ is to stimulate active absorption of calcium (and phosphate) by the intestine. Thus, the major event in vitamin D deficiency is decreased gut calcium absorption, resulting in decreased plasma calcium. In children, the newly formed bone protein matrix fails to be calcified normally because of the low plasma calcium, leading to the disease **rickets.**

In addition to its effect on intestinal calcium absorption, $1,25\text{-}(OH)_2D_3$ also significantly enhances bone resorption. The mechanism underlying this effect is unclear but may involve a facilitation by $1,25\text{-}(OH)_2D_3$ of the bone resorption effect exerted by parathyroid hormone. Finally, $1,25\text{-}(OH)_2D_3$ can also stimulate the renal-tubular reabsorption of calcium (and phosphate).

The blood concentration of $1,25\text{-}(OH)_2D_3$ is subject to physiological control. The major control point is the second hydroxylation step, the one that occurs in the kidneys. This step is stimulated by parathyroid hormone, a phenomenon that is highly adaptive because it provides a mechanism for simultaneously altering the levels of these hormones in the same direction. Thus, a low plasma calcium concentration stimulates the secretion of parathyroid hormone, which in turn enhances the production of $1,25\text{-}(OH)_2D_3$, and both hormones contribute to the restoration of the plasma calcium to normal (Fig. 10-2).[5]

Calcitonin

Calcitonin is a peptide hormone secreted by cells within the thyroid gland that surround, but are completely distinct from, the thyroid follicles. The calcitonin-secreting cells are called, therefore, **parafollicular cells.** Calcitonin can lower plasma calcium, primarily by inhibiting bone resorption. Its secretion is controlled, in part, directly by the calcium concentration of the plasma supplying the thyroid gland; increased calcium causes increased calcitonin secretion. Thus, this system has been suspected of constituting another feedback control over plasma calcium concentration. However, its overall contribution to calcium homeostasis is very minor compared with that of parathyroid hormone and $1,25\text{-}(OH)_2D_3$. Indeed, thyroidectomized persons with no detectable plasma calcitonin have no significant alteration in their plasma calcium concentration. Accordingly, emphasis has shifted away from calcitonin as a regulator of plasma calcium and toward its possible roles in regulating other physiological activities.[6]

Other Hormones

Parathyroid hormone and $1,25\text{-}(OH)_2D_3$ are the major hormones that participate in *homeostatic* responses to changes in calcium balance. However, several other hormones do influence calcium, so that changes in their rates of secretion can produce calcium imbalances. Thus, for example, high levels of cortisol can induce negative calcium balance by depressing gut absorption of calcium while increasing its renal excretion. To take another example, growth hormone also increases urinary calcium excretion, but it simultaneously increases gut absorption; the net effect of these counterbalancing influences of growth hormone is usually a positive calcium balance.

OVERVIEW OF RENAL PHOSPHATE HANDLING

The renal handling of phosphate has been mentioned several times in this chapter and elsewhere in the book but almost always in the context of other topics, such as sodium reabsorption or urine acidification. This section reviews certain key aspects of renal phosphate handling since control of urinary phosphate excretion is a major pathway for the homeostatic regulation of total-body phosphate balance (Fig. 10-3).

Approximately 5 to 10 percent of plasma phosphate is protein-bound, so that 90 to 95 percent is filterable at the renal corpuscle. Normally, approximately 75 percent of this filtered phosphate is actively reabsorbed, almost entirely in the proximal tubule (in cotransport with sodium).[7]

As with other substances handled by filtration and tubular reabsorption, the rate of phosphate excretion can be changed by altering the mass filtered per unit time and/or the mass reabsorbed per unit time. Indeed, even relatively small increases in plasma phosphate concentration (and, hence, filtered load) can produce relatively large increases in phosphate excretion. This occurs when plasma phosphate concentration increases as a result of increased dietary phosphate intake.

But changes in filtered load are not the major reason that phosphate excretion increases or decreases homeostatically in response to altered dietary intake. Tubular reabsorption also changes. A diet low in phosphate induces, over time, an increase in the rate of phosphate reabsorption; a diet high in phosphate does just the opposite. Changes in the secretion and, hence, plasma

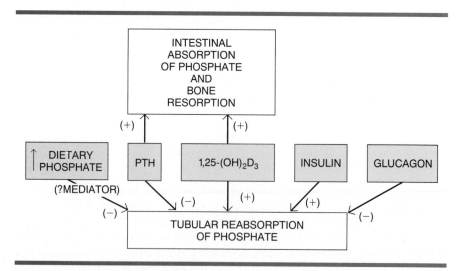

Fig. 10-3 Effects of hormones and dietary phosphate on phosphate movements. (+) denotes a stimulation, and (−) an inhibition. Moreover, each (+) will tend to raise plasma phosphate concentration, whereas each (−) will tend to lower it.

concentrations of parathyroid hormone and $1,25\text{-}(OH)_2D_3$ may play minor roles[8] but the major input remains unknown.

To reiterate, changes in parathyroid hormone [and $1,25\text{-}(OH)_2D_3$] do not mediate the homeostatic association between dietary phosphate and tubular phosphate reabsorption. Nevertheless, as we have seen, whenever parathyroid hormone is increased or decreased, tubular phosphate reabsorption is powerfully inhibited or stimulated, respectively. Other hormones, too, are known to alter phosphate reabsorption; e.g., inulin increases it and glucagon decreases it.[9]

Study questions: 69 to 71

NOTES

[1]The electrochemical forces are (1) a proximal *concentration* difference created by proximal water reabsorption, and (2) the lumen-positive *electrical potential difference* in the middle-to-late proximal tubule and the thick ascending limb. As we have seen, the creation of both these forces requires sodium reabsorption. (See Costanzo and Windhager in Suggested Readings.)

[2]An interesting indication of the differences in reabsorption of calcium and sodium in the distal convoluted tubule is the fact that diuretics that inhibit sodium reabsorption by this tubular segment facilitate calcium reabsorption by it. In contrast, diuretics that act mainly in the proximal tubule and/or thick ascending limb of Henle's loop inhibit reabsorption of both ions.

[3]Parathyroid hormone actually *inhibits* calcium reabsorption by the proximal tubule, mainly because it inhibits sodium reabsorption (see Chapters 7 and 9), but the *overall* tubular effect of this hormone is to increase calcium reabsorption because the more distal stimulatory effect predominates.

[4]Another candidate to join these four was mentioned in Chapter 9—parathyroid hormone's inhibition of proximal-tubular hydrogen-ion secretion (via an effect on the luminal-membrane Na/H countertransporter) and, thereby, bicarbonate reabsorption. The result of this effect is increased extracellular fluid hydrogen-ion concentration (acidosis), which is known to displace calcium from plasma protein (as described in the text) and from bone. Thus, free plasma calcium concentration rises. Whether this effect of parathyroid hormone is really important at physiological plasma levels of the hormone is still not settled.

[5]Parathyroid hormone is not the only modulator of $1,25\text{-}(OH)_2D_3$ formation by the kidneys. Phosphate is another important one, decreased plasma phosphate stimulating formation. This is adaptive in terms of phosphate homeostasis: Decreased plasma phosphate concentration stimulates formation of $1,25\text{-}(OH)_2D_3$, which then enhances phosphate release from bone, absorption from the gut, and reabsorption by the renal tubules, with a resulting compensatory increase in plasma phosphate. Many other possible inputs are presently being studied. For example, it is likely that estrogen and prolactin also stimulate renal formation of $1,25\text{-}(OH)_2D_3$. This would be adaptive in

increasing gut absorption of calcium and phosphate during pregnancy. Insulin-like growth factor 1 also stimulates renal formation of 1,25-$(OH)_2D_3$, and this may play an important role during growth.

[6]See Austin and Heath in Suggested Readings.

[7]There is probably also some small degree of phosphate reabsorption in sites beyond the proximal tubule. There is no conclusive evidence for significant tubular secretion of phosphate, although this remains controversial.

[8]Parathyroid hormone secretion is decreased when plasma phosphate decreases, because the latter causes a rise in plasma ionized calcium concentration; the lowered parathyroid hormone would result in greater phosphate reabsorption. Despite the decrease in parathyroid hormone, the formation of 1,25-$(OH)_2D_3$ is increased when plasma phosphate decreases because, as described in note 5, phosphate is an important stimulator of the 1-hydroxylation step in the formation of 1,25-$(OH)_2D_3$.

[9]See Dennis, and Berndt and Knox in Suggested Readings.

As emphasized in the Preface, these questions do not cover the material of this book systematically or comprehensively; that is the function of the objectives at the beginning of each chapter. Rather, they provide practice and additional feedback in certain areas, particularly those that commonly give some difficulty.

Q-1 The difference between superficial and juxtamedullary nephrons is that the former have their glomeruli in the cortex whereas the glomeruli of the latter arise in the medulla. True or false?

A-1 False. All glomeruli are in the cortex. See text for description.

Q-2 When a patient is given a drug that inhibits angiotensin-converting enzyme, there is little physiological effect because the decrement in angiotensin II is compensated by the simultaneous rise in angiotensin I. True or false?

A-2 False. Angiotensin II is much more potent than angiotensin I.

Q-3 Substance *T* is present in the urine. Does this *prove* that it is filterable at the glomerulus?

A-3 No. It is a possibility, but there is another: Substance *T* may be secreted by the tubules.

Q-4 Substance *V* is not normally present in the urine. Does this *prove* that it is neither filtered nor secreted?

A-4 No. It is a possibility, but there is another: *V* may be filtered and/or secreted, but all the *V* entering the lumen via these routes may be completely reabsorbed.

Q-5 The concentration of calcium in Bowman's capsule is 3 mmol/L, whereas its plasma concentration is 5 mmol/L. How do you explain this?

A-5 Approximately 40 percent of the calcium in plasma is bound to proteins and so is not filterable.

Q-6 The concentration of glucose in plasma is 100 mg/100 ml and the GFR is 125 ml/min. How much glucose is filtered per minute?

A-6 125 mg/min. The amount of *any* substance filtered per unit time is given by the product of the GFR and the filterable plasma concentration of the substance, in this case, 125 ml/min × 100 mg/100 ml.

Q-7 A protein has a molecular weight of 30,000 and a plasma concentration of 100 mg/L. The GFR is 100 L/day. How much of this protein is filtered per day?

A-7 No exact value can be calculated from these data because the concentration of the protein in the glomerular filtrate is not known. The molecular weight is high enough so that some "sieving" would occur but low enough so that the restriction would not be total.

Q-8 A drug is noted to cause a decrease in GFR. What might the drug be doing?
A-8 **a** Constricting glomerular mesangial cells and, hence, reducing K_f
      b Lowering arterial pressure and, hence, P_{GC}
      c Constricting the afferent arteriole and, hence, reducing P_{GC}
      d Dilating the efferent arteriole and, hence, reducing P_{GC}
      e Causing obstruction somewhere in the urinary system and, hence, increasing P_{BC}
      f Increasing plasma albumin concentration and, hence, Π_{GC}
      g Decreasing the amount of blood flow to the kidneys, resulting in a steeper rise of Π_{GC} along the length of the glomerular capillaries

Q-9 A drug is noted to cause an increase in GFR with no change in net filtration pressure. What must the drug be doing?
A-9 It must be increasing K_f, i.e., changing the hydraulic permeability of the gomerular membranes and/or the surface area available for filtration.

Q-10 A person is given a drug that dilates the afferent arteriole and constricts the efferent arteriole by the same amounts. Assuming no other actions of the drug, what happens to this person's GFR, RBF, and filtration fraction?
A-10 RBF will show no change since the drug has no effect on *total* renal vascular resistance. GFR will increase, because of a large increase in P_{GC}. Filtration fraction will, therefore, increase. (Now back up and think a bit more about the GFR: Since filtration fraction increases, there will be a larger than average rise in Π_{GC} along the glomeruli, and this will offset some of the GFR-increasing effect of the increased P_{GC}; therefore, GFR will not go up as much proportionately as the P_{GC}.)

Q-11 During a dog experiment, a clamp around the renal artery is partially tightened to reduce renal arterial pressure from a mean of 120 mmHg to 80 mmHg. How much do you predict RBF will change?
      a 33 percent decrease
      b Zero
      c 5 to 10 percent decrease
      d 33 percent increase
A-11 *c*. Autoregulation prevents the RBF from decreasing in direct proportion to mean arterial pressure, but autoregulation is not 100 percent complete.

Q-12 A patient suffers a hemorrhage that drops the mean arterial pressure by 25 percent. What do you predict happens to the GFR and RBF?
      a Almost no change
      b A fairly large decrease in RBF, and a smaller decrease in GFR
A-12 *b*. If you answered *a*, you probably assumed that autoregulation would prevent any significant change. This is wrong because the drop in pressure reflexly stimulates increased sympathetic tone to the kidney and increased plasma angiotensin II. (See text for the reason the GFR change is less than the RBF change.)

Q-13 A normal dog is given a drug that inhibits sodium chloride reabsorption by the proximal tubule. GFR decreases within seconds to a particular value and then slowly decreases even more over the next 2 h. Why?

A-13 The immediate decrease in GFR is due to tubuloglomerular feedback; the more delayed additional decrease is due to reflexly increased sympathetic outflow to the kidney and increased angiotensin II, both triggered reflexly by the progressive diuretic-induced depletion of bodily sodium and water.

Q-14 In the situation described in Q-12, what would happen to RBF (relative to its value following the hemorrhage) if the hemorrhaged person were given a drug that blocks synthesis of prostaglandins?
  a Increase
  b Remain the same
  c Decrease

A-14 *c.* Increased sympathetic outflow and increased angiotensin II induce the synthesis of vasodilator prostaglandins; the drug would prevent this and, hence, eliminate the usual prostaglandin-dependent opposition to renal vasoconstriction.

Q-15 A dog is subjected to a mild hemorrhage; its mean arterial pressure decreases slightly, and its plasma renin concentration increases markedly. It is then given a drug that blocks β-adrenergic receptors. Its plasma renin decreases back toward the normal (prehemorrhage) values but remains somewhat elevated. Why?

A-15 Most of the stimulus for increased renin release in this situation occurs through the renal sympathetic nerves and epinephrine, which act directly on the granular cells via β-adrenergic receptors. Some stimulus remains, however, via the intrarenal baroreceptor and macula densa.

Q-16 A normal person is given a drug that blocks angiotensin-converting enzyme. What happens to renin secretion?

A-16 It increases. Angiotensin II exerts a potent inhibitory effect on renin secretion; therefore, eliminating angiotensin II relieves this inhibition, resulting in more renin secretion.

Q-17 The hospital lab reports that your patient's creatinine clearance is 120 g/day. This value is
  a Normal
  b Significantly below normal
  c Nonsense

A-17 *c.* Clearance units are volume per time, not mass per time.

Q-18 The following test results were obtained on specimens from a person over a 2-h period during infusion of inulin and PAH:

$$\text{Total urine vol} = 0.14 \text{ L}$$
$$U_{In} = 100 \text{ mg/100 ml}$$
$$P_{In} = 1 \text{ mg/100 ml}$$
$$U_{urea} = 220 \text{ mmol/L}$$
$$P_{urea} = 5 \text{ mmol/L}$$
$$U_{PAH} = 700 \text{ mg/L}$$
$$P_{PAH} = 2 \text{ mg/L}$$
$$\text{Hematocrit} = 0.40$$

What are the clearances of inulin, urea, and PAH? What is the effective renal plasma flow (ERPF)? What is the effective renal blood flow (ERBF)? How much urea is reabsorbed? How much PAH is secreted (assuming no PAH reabsorption and complete filterability of PAH)?

A-18

$$C_{In} = \frac{U_{In}\, V}{P_{In}}$$

$$= \frac{100 \text{ mg}/100 \text{ ml} \times 0.14 \text{ L}/2 \text{ h}}{1 \text{ mg}/100 \text{ ml}}$$

$$= 14.0 \text{ L}/2 \text{ h; this is the GFR}$$

$$C_{urea} = \frac{U_{urea}\, V}{P_{urea}}$$

$$= \frac{220 \text{ mmol/L} \times 0.14 \text{ L}/2 \text{ h}}{5 \text{ mmol/L}}$$

$$= 6.16 \text{ L}/2 \text{ h}$$

$$C_{PAH} = \frac{U_{PAH}\, V}{P_{PAH}}$$

$$= \frac{700 \text{ mg/L} \times 0.14 \text{ L}/2 \text{ h}}{2 \text{ mg/L}}$$

$$= 49.0 \text{ L}/2 \text{ h}$$

$$\text{ERPF} = 49.0 \text{ L}/2 \text{ h}$$

$$\text{ERBF} = 81.7 \text{ L}/2 \text{ h}$$

$$\text{Reabsorbed urea} = \text{filtered urea} - \text{excreted urea}$$

$$= (14.0 \text{ L}/2 \text{ h} \times 5 \text{ mmol/L})$$
$$-(220 \text{ mmol/L} \times 0.14 \text{ L}/2 \text{ h})$$
$$= 39.2 \text{ mmol}/2 \text{ h}$$

$$\text{PAH secreted} = \text{PAH excreted} - \text{PAH filtered}$$

$$= (700 \text{ mg/L} \times 0.14 \text{ L}/2 \text{ h})$$
$$-(2 \text{ mg/L} \times 14.0 \text{ L}/2 \text{ h})$$
$$= 98.0 \text{ mg}/2 \text{ h} - 28.0 \text{ g}/2 \text{ h}$$
$$= 70.0 \text{ mg}/2 \text{ h}$$

Q-19 An increase in the plasma concentration of inulin causes which of the following in the renal clearance of inulin?

a Increase
b Decrease
c No change

A-19 c. $C_{In} = U_{In}V/P_{In}$. When P_{In} increases, there is no change in C_{In} because U_{In} rises by an identical amount. In other words, the mass of inulin filtered and excreted increases, but the volume of plasma supplying this inulin, i.e., completely cleared of inulin, is unaltered.

Q-20 The clearance of substance A is less than that simultaneously determined for inulin. Give three possible explanations.

A-20 1. Substance A is a large molecule poorly filtered at the glomerulus.
2. Substance A is bound, at least in part, to plasma protein.
3. Substance A is reabsorbed.

Q-21 The clearance of substance B is greater than the simultaneously determined clearance for inulin. What is the only possible explanation for this?

A-21 Substance B is secreted by the tubules.

Q-22 List in order of decreasing renal clearance the following substances:
Glucose
Urea
Sodium
Inulin
Creatinine
PAH
A-22 PAH
Creatinine
Inulin
Urea
Sodium
Glucose

Q-23 The following test results were obtained during a clearance experiment.
$$U_{In} = 50 \text{ mg/L}$$
$$P_{In} = 1 \text{ mg/L}$$
$$V = 2 \text{ ml/min}$$
$$U_{Na} = 75 \text{ mmol/L}$$
$$P_{Na} = 150 \text{ mmol/L}$$
What is the fractional excretion (FE) of sodium?
A-23 0.01.
$$FE_{Na} = \frac{\text{mass Na excreted}}{\text{mass Na filtered}} = \frac{U_{Na} \, V}{GFR \times P_{Na}} = \frac{U_{Na} \, V}{C_{In} \times P_{Na}}$$
$$= \frac{75 \text{ mmol/L} \times 2 \text{ ml/min}}{100 \text{ ml/min} \times 150 \text{ mmol/L}}$$
$$= 0.01$$
This means that only 1 percent of the filtered sodium was excreted; i.e., 99 percent was reabsorbed.

Q-24 During a micropuncture experiment, a sample of tubular fluid (TF) was obtained from the end of the proximal tubule and its inulin concentration was found to be twice as high as the concentration in plasma, i.e., $TF_{In}/P_{In} = 2$. How much water was reabsorbed by the proximal tubule?
A-24 Fifty percent of the water that was originally filtered. Since inulin is neither reabsorbed nor secreted, its rise in concentration along the tubule is due entirely to water reabsorption and can, therefore, be used to calculate the extent of water reabsorption.

Q-25 A month after 80 percent of the nephrons are destroyed, what will the blood urea concentration be, assuming it was 5 mmol/L before the disease occurred?
a 25 mmol/L
b 5 mmol/L
c 6 mmol/L
d Continuously rising
e Not calculable unless it is assumed that the patient's protein intake did not change as a result of the disease

A-25 *e.* If one assumes constant protein intake, 25 mmol/L would have been the correct answer since total filtered urea could be restored to normal at this point [25(0.2 × 180) = 5 × 180]. However, had protein intake been reduced by 50 percent, plasma urea would stabilize at 12.5 mmol/L since only 50 percent as much urea would be produced.

Q-26 There is a net movement of anionic phosphate across the luminal membrane into the tubular cells even though cytosolic phosphate concentration is higher than luminal phosphate concentration and there is a cytosol-negative potential difference across the luminal membrane. Does this prove that the phosphate movement is driven by the direct input of energy from splitting ATP?

A-26 No. It proves that the movement is active, but it could be a secondary active transport (and, in fact, is).

Q-27 You are trying to measure the reabsorptive T_m for glucose in a patient. You plan to calculate glucose reabsorption $[(GFR \times P_G) - (U_G \times V)]$ as you raise plasma glucose stepwise by infusion. You stop the test when glucose first appears in the urine, assuming that the reabsorptive rate at this time equals the T_m. Is this correct?

A-27 No. Glucose starts to appear in the urine *before* the T_m for all nephrons has been reached. Therefore, if you had continued to raise plasma glucose, the reabsorptive rate would have increased some more. You can be certain the T_m has been reached only when the reabsorptive rate remains constant despite another increment in plasma glucose.

Q-28 If 50 percent of a person's nephrons were destroyed, which of the following compounds would be likely to show increased blood concentration?
  a Urea
  b Creatinine
  c Uric acid
  d Most amino acids
  e Glucose

A-28 *a, b, c.* These waste products are all normally excreted in large amounts; a decreased GFR would cause their plasma concentrations to increase until the filtered load was increased enough to reestablish normal excretion. In contrast, the reabsorption T_ms for glucose, amino acids, and many other organic compounds that are not waste products are usually so high as to prevent significant excretion. Accordingly, their plasma concentrations are virtually independent of renal function, i.e., the kidneys do not participate in the setting of their plasma concentrations.

Q-29 The concentration of urea in urine is always much higher than the concentration in plasma. Is this because the overall tubular handling of urea is secretion?

A-29 No. The overall tubular handling of urea is reabsorption. The reason urinary urea concentration is higher than that of plasma is that relatively more water has been reabsorbed than urea, thereby concentrating the urea in the tubule.

Q-30 If the concentration of protein in the glomerular filtrate was 0.005 g/100 ml and none was reabsorbed, how much protein would be excreted per day (assuming a normal GFR)?

A-30 9 g.

$$\text{Excreted} = \text{filtered} - \text{reabsorbed}$$
$$= (0.05 \, \text{g/L} \times 180 \, \text{L/day}) - 0$$
$$= 9 \, \text{g/day}$$

Q-31 A drug has been found to increase uric acid excretion. Give at least three ways it might act.

A-31 1. Increase uric acid synthesis $\rightarrow$ increased plasma uric acid $\rightarrow$ increased filtration of uric acid
2. Stimulation of secretion of uric acid
3. Inhibition of reabsorption of uric acid

Q-32 If you wished to increase your patient's excretion of quinine, a weak organic base, what change in urinary pH would you try to induce?

A-32 Decreased pH. This would convert more of the quinine to its charged form and prevent its passive reabsorption.

Q-33 In the steady state, what is the amount of sodium chloride excreted daily in the urine by a normal person ingesting 12 g of sodium chloride per day?
a 12 g/day
b Less than 12 g/day

A-33 *b.* Urinary excretion in the steady state must be less than ingested sodium chloride by an amount equal to that lost in the sweat and feces. This is normally quite small, less than 1 g/day, so that urine execretion in this case equals approximately 11 g/day.

Q-34 A person's plasma sodium concentration is 144 mmol/L; inulin clearance, 120 ml/min; urine volume, 36 ml in 30 min; and urine sodium concentration, 200 mmol/L. What percentage of filtered sodium is excreted?

A-34 1.4 percent.

$$\text{Filtered Na}^+ = 144 \, \text{mmol/L} \times 0.12 \, \text{L/min}$$
$$= 17.28 \, \text{mmol/min}$$
$$\text{Excreted Na}^+ = 0.036 \, \text{L/30 min} \times 200 \, \text{mmol/L}$$
$$= 0.24 \, \text{mmol/min}$$
$$\% \frac{\text{excreted}}{\text{filtered}} = \frac{0.24}{17.28} \times 100 = 1.4\%$$

Q-35 In chronic renal disease, plasma urea may become markedly elevated. Under such circumstances urea will act as an osmotic diuretic. What does this do to sodium, chloride, and water excretion?

A-35 Sodium, chloride, and water excretion will all increase.

Q-36 **a** Complete inhibition of active sodium and chloride transport by the thick ascending limb of Henle's loop would virtually eliminate the ability to excrete a concentrated urine. True or false?
b Increasing the passive permeability of the thick ascending limb of Henle's loop to sodium and chloride would reduce the maximal concentrating ability of the kidney. True or false?
c Active reabsorption of sodium and chloride by the descending thin limb of Henle's loop is a component of the countercurrent multiplier system. True or false?

A-36 a. True.

      b. True. The gradient between ascending loop and interstitium at any *horizontal level* would be decreased; therefore the gradient from top to bottom would be decreased.

      c. False. There is no reabsorption of sodium or chloride by the descending thin limb of Henle's loop.

Q-37 A normal experimental animal is given a drug, and a sample of tubular fluid (TF) is later collected by micropuncture from the end of the proximal convoluted tubule along with a plasma (P) sample. The TF/P ratio for inulin is 1.5, and for sodium, 0.99. Has the drug inhibited, stimulated, or done nothing to proximal sodium reabsorption?

A-37 Inhibited it. The inulin data reveal that only 30 percent of filtered water has been reabsorbed. Since TF/P for sodium is essentially unity (the normal value for proximal fluid), this means that only 30 percent of the filtered sodium was reabsorbed, a value far below normal. If you are having trouble understanding this relatively difficult question, look at note 3 in Chapter 3.

Q-38 True or false:

      a Net reabsorption of sodium occurs in the thick ascending limb of Henle's loop.

      b Net reabsorption of water occurs in the descending thin limb of Henle's loop.

      c Net reabsorption of water occurs in the collecting ducts in the presence of ADH.

      d Net bulk flow of interstitial fluid into the vasa recta occurs.

A-38 All are true. The last may have given you trouble. The fact is that the vasa recta act as countercurrent exchangers to eliminate net overall *diffusion* of sodium and water into or out of the vasa recta by balancing any net movements in the descending vessels with opposite ones in the ascending. Thus, net diffusional movements are minimal, but normal capillary *bulk-flow* must still be occurring, or otherwise the sodium and water reabsorbed from the loops of Henle and collecting ducts would not be carried away.

Q-39 A drug is given that blocks all sodium channels and transporters in the luminal membrane all along the tubule but does not act on the Na,K-ATPase pumps in the basolateral membrane. What happens to sodium reabsorption?

A-39 It ceases completely. Even though the active step is not altered by the drug, there will be no sodium entering the cell to be acted on by the pumps.

Q-40 A drug is given that blocks all Na,K-ATPase in the tubule. Would this eliminate chloride reabsorption in all nephron segments?

A-40 Chloride reabsorption would be blocked everywhere except the cortical collecting duct. The active process for chloride in this latter segment is by countertransport with bicarbonate and is sodium-independent.

Q-41 In an experiment a dog's rate of glomerular filtration of sodium in an isolated pump-perfused kidney is found to be 15 mmol/min.

      a How much sodium do you predict remains in the tubule at the end of the proximal tubule?

      b Its GFR is suddenly increased by 33 percent. How much sodium now is left at the end of the proximal tubule?

A-41 a. 5 mmol/min. Approximately two-thirds of filtered sodium is reabsorbed by the proximal tubule.

          b. 6.6 mmol/min. Filtered sodium rises from 15 to 20 mmol/min. Glomerulo-tubular balance maintains fractional sodium reabsorption at approximately two-thirds of the filtered load.

Q-42 Normally aldosterone controls the reabsorption of approximately 33 g of sodium chloride per day. If a patient loses 100 percent of adrenal function, will 33 g of sodium chloride be excreted per day indefinitely?

A-42 No. As soon as the person starts to become sodium-deficient as a result of the increased sodium excretion, the usual sodium-retaining reflexes will be set into motion. They will, of course, be unable to raise aldosterone secretion, but they will lower GFR and alter the other factors that influence tubular sodium reab-sorption to compensate at least partially for the decreased aldosterone-depen-dent sodium reabsorption.

Q-43 What happens to sodium excretion during quiet standing?

A-43 It decreases. Because of venous pooling of blood and increased filtration of fluid across the leg capillaries, quiet standing causes an effective decrease in plasma volume, which triggers all the described inputs leading to decreased sodium excretion (decreased GFR and increased tubular reabsorption).

Q-44 A patient has just suffered a severe hemorrhage and the plasma protein concen-tration is normal. (Not enough time has elapsed for interstitial fluid to move into the plasma.) Does this mean that the peritubular-capillary oncotic pressure is also normal?

A-44 No. It will probably be above normal because of increased filtration fraction secondary to renal arteriolar constriction mediated by the renal sympathetic nerves and angiotensin II.

Q-45 If the right renal artery becomes abnormally constricted, what will happen to renin secretion by it and by the left kidney?

A-45 The right kidney will have increased secretion because of decreased renal per-fusion pressure acting via the intrarenal baroceptor and decreased flow to the macula densa. This increased secretion will result in elevated systemic arterial angiotensin II and arterial blood pressure, both of which will inhibit renin secretion from the left kidney.

Q-46 A patient with leaky glomeruli but normal tubules loses protein in the urine and, therefore, has a plasma albumin of 2.5 g/100ml. Virtually all sodium ingested is retained (i.e., urinary excretion of sodium is close to zero) and the patient is becoming edematous. What is the stimulus for renal sodium retention in this case since total extracellular volume is clearly greater than normal?

A-46 Because of the low plasma albumin, *plasma volume* is decreased as a result of the abnormal balance of forces across capillaries. This decreased plasma volume initiates sodium-retaining reflexes just as if the plasma volume had been de-creased by diarrhea, a burn, etc. The retained fluid does not restore the plasma volume to normal, however, but merely filters into the interstitium, where it increases the edema. Interestingly, tubular sodium reabsorption is increased in this state despite the fact that peritubular-capillary protein concentration is almost certainly lower than normal, which should reduce tubular sodium reabsorption. A reflexly increased aldosterone level is certainly important in stimulating sodium reabsorption and overriding this effect of the low protein. Changes in renal hemodynamics may also be important.

Q-47 A patient is suffering from primary hyperaldosteronism, i.e., increased secretion of aldosterone, usually caused by an aldosterone-producing adrenal tumor. Is plasma renin concentration higher or lower than normal?

A-47 Lower. The increased aldosterone causes positive sodium balance, which reflexly inhibits renin secretion. Thus, one observes high plasma aldosterone and low plasma renin—a strong tip-off to the presence of the disease since in almost all other situations renin and aldosterone change in the same direction (because the renin-angiotensin system is the major control of aldosterone secretion).

Q-48 Any agent that increases sodium and water excretion is called a *diuretic* (even though *natriuretic* is probably a better term). List possible mechanisms of the actions of these drugs.

A-48 1. They increase GFR either by raising blood pressure or by dilating renal afferent arterioles.
2. They cause hemodynamic changes that increase renal interstitial hydraulic pressure.
3. They directly inhibit the active-transport system for sodium, e.g., by blocking Na,K-ATPase.
4. They directly block the Na,K,2Cl cotransporter in the thick ascending limb of Henle's loop.
5. They directly block the Na,Cl cotransporter in the distal convoluted tubule.
6. They inhibit sodium-hydrogen-ion countertransport.
7. They inhibit secretion of renin, the formation of angiotensin II, or the action of angiotensin II on the adrenal cortex.
8. They block the action of aldosterone.
9. They act as an osmotic diuretic by their osmotic contribution.
   This list is by no means exhaustive but does include the major clinically useful types of diuretics.

Q-49 A person is given a drug that dilates both the afferent and efferent arterioles. Assuming no other action of the drug, what will happen to the percent of filtered sodium that this person's proximal tubule reabsorbs?

A-49 It will decrease. This question focuses on the effect of renal interstitial hydraulic pressure (RIHP) on proximal sodium reabsorption and is simply the exact opposite of the situation produced by stimulation of the renal sympathetic nerves: (1) The person has a large decrease in total renal vascular resistance and so will have a large increase in peritubular-capillary hydraulic pressure (P_{PC}). (2) There is also a large increase in RBF and either no change or a small increase in GFR (P_{GC} remains relatively unchanged but Π_{GC} rises less than normally because of the large rise in RBF); hence filtration fraction goes down, which causes a decrease in peritubular-capillary oncotic pressure (Π_{PC}). Both the increased P_{PC} and the decreased Π_{PC} raise RIHP, which reduces proximal sodium and water reabsorption. (The question was phrased in terms of "percentage of filtered sodium" reabsorbed so that you could ignore glomerulotubular balance in thinking about the answer. In other words, to the extent that GFR rises in this situation, that alone would, by glomerulotubular balance, tend to raise *absolute* sodium reabsorption but not the percentage of filtered sodium reabsorbed.)

Q-50 A normal subject loses 2 L of isotonic salt solution because of diarrhea. He or she simultaneously drinks 2 L of pure water. What happens to
  a Extracellular fluid volume
  b Body fluid osmolarity
  c Renin and aldosterone secretion
  d ADH secretion

A-50 a and b. Extracellular volume and osmolarity both decrease. The entire 2 L of solution was lost from the extracellular compartment since it was isotonic. (Therefore, osmolarity did not change, and no water moved into or out of cells.) The 2 L of ingested pure water is distributed throughout the bodily water, only about one-third remaining in the extracellular fluid. Moreover, the addition of pure water lowers the osmolarity.
  c. This increases because of reflexes induced by the decreased extracellular volume.
  d. We cannot predict for certain, but it probably decreases. The decreased extracellular volume reflexly stimulates ADH secretion, but the reduced osmolarity should inhibit it via the hypothalamic osmoreceptors. The osmoreceptor input usually predominates during such "conflicts" unless the extracellular volume depletion is very large.

Q-51 A person excretes 2 L of urine having an osmolarity of 600 mOsm/L. As a result, does bodily fluid osmolarity *increase* or *decrease*?

A-51 It decreases. He or she has excreted 2 L × 600 mOsm/L = 1200 mOsm total solute and 2 L water. Two liters of normal bodily fluids contain 2 L × 300 mOsm/L = 600 mOsm solutes. Accordingly, he or she has excreted relatively more solute than water, compared to the normal proportions in the bodily fluids. This will reduce the bodily fluid osmolarity.

Q-52 A person excretes 3 L of urine having an osmolarity of 150 mOsm/L. As a result, does bodily fluid osmolarity *increase* or *decrease*?

A-52 It increases. He or she has excreted 3 L × 150 mOsm/L = 450 mOsm total solute, and 3 L water have been excreted. This amount of solute is contained in 450 mOsm ÷ 300 mOsm/L = 1.5 L normal body fluid. Therefore, he or she has excreted relatively more water than solute, compared to the normal proportions in the bodily fluids.

Q-53 What are the major renal sites of action of the following hormones?
  Aldosterone
  ADH
  Renin
  Epinephrine
  Angiotensin II

A-53 Aldosterone: Cortical collecting duct (principal cells)
  ADH: Cortical and medullary collecting ducts (principal cells)
  Renin: No renal site of action
  Epinephrine: Renal arterioles, JG apparatus, and renal tubules (mainly proximal tubule)

Angiotensin II: Renal arterioles and renal tubules (mainly proximal tubule)

Q-54 What are the major controls of aldosterone secretion?
A-54 1. Angiotensin II
2. ACTH
3. Plasma potassium concentration

Q-55 What are the major controls of renin secretion?
A-55 1. Afferent-arteriolar pressure (intrarenal baroreceptor)
2. Sodium chloride load to the macula densa
3. Activity of renal sympathetic nerves
4. Angiotensin II

Q-56 What are the major controls of ADH secretion?
A-56 1. Bodily fluid osmolarity via hypothalamic osmoreceptors
2. Plasma volume (via cardiovascular baroreceptors)

Q-57 Control of potassium excretion is achieved mainly by regulating the rate of which of the following?
a Potassium filtration
b Potassium reabsorption
c Potassium secretion
A-57 *c.*

Q-58 A person in previously normal potassium balance maintains neurotic hyperventilation for several days. During this period what happens to potassium balance?
A-58 It becomes negative. The hyperventilation causes alkalosis, which in turn induces increased secretion of potassium (probably because of an alkalosis-induced elevation of renal-tubular cell potassium concentration).

Q-59 A patient has a tumor in the adrenal that continuously secretes large quantities of aldosterone (primary hyperaldosteronism). Is the rate of potassium excretion normal, high, or low?
A-59 High. The increased aldosterone stimulates potassium secretion and, thereby, excretion. Moreover, once enough sodium has been retained to increase GFR and to cause partial inhibition of proximal reabsorption, the increased delivery of fluid to the cortical collecting duct further enhances potassium secretion. There is no potassium escape similar to the sodium escape from aldosterone.

Q-60 A patient with severe congestive heart failure is secreting large quantities of aldosterone. Is the rate of potassium excretion normal, high, or low?
A-60 Relatively normal. You may well have answered "high," assuming that the increased aldosterone would stimulate potassium secretion, as in the previous question. However, this effect is more than balanced by the fact that the patient has a decrease in flow of fluid into the cortical collecting duct (because of decreased GFR and increased proximal and loop reabsorption); recall that potassium secretion is impaired when the amount of fluid flowing through the cortical collecting duct is reduced. This explains why patients with the diseases of secondary hyperaldosteronism with edema do not lose large quantities of potassium, whereas patients with primary hyperaldosteronism do.

Q-61 A person with congestive heart failure has an elevated plasma aldosterone and is retaining sodium. She has a normal plasma pH. She is started on diuretics that block sodium reabsorption in the thick ascending limb of Henle's loop, and her plasma pH increases after a few days, i.e., she develops metabolic alkalosis. What is the mechanism?

A-61 Before receiving the diuretic her potassium balance was probably normal because the stimulatory effect of the high aldosterone on potassium secretion was being offset by the inhibitory effect of the low collecting-duct flow (caused by decreased GFR and increased proximal sodium reabsorption) typical of persons with congestive heart failure (question 60). The diuretic, by increasing collecting-duct flow, will add to the stimulatory effect of aldosterone and cause a marked increase in potassium secretion. This, in turn, can cause potassium depletion, which will then synergize with the high aldosterone to cause an inappropriate increase in tubular hydrogen-ion secretion and ammonium production. Thus, the kidneys will create a metabolic alkalosis by contributing too much new bicarbonate to the blood.

Q-62 Give three reasons why osmotic diuresis (as, for example, in uncontrolled diabetic ketoacidosis) enhances potassium excretion.

A-62 1. It inhibits potassium reabsorption by the proximal tubule.
2. It increases fluid delivery to the cortical collecting duct, resulting in increased potassium secretion.
3. It causes sodium depletion, which increases aldosterone secretion (via the renin-angiotensin system), and this hormone stimulates potassium secretion.

Q-63 A patient is observed to excrete 2 L of alkaline (pH = 7.6) urine having a bicarbonate concentration of 28 mmol/L. The rate of titratable-acid excretion is
a 56 mmol
b Negative
c Cannot tell without data for ammonium

A-63 *b*. If the urine has a pH greater than 7.4, clearly there is no titratable acid (t.a.) excreted; indeed, there is negative t.a. excretion. Ammonium does not contribute to t.a. and may be ignored in the calculation of t.a.

Q-64 The following data are obtained for a subject:
$$C_{In} = 170 \text{ L/day}$$
$$P_{HCO_3^-} = 25 \text{ mmol/L}$$
$$U_{HCO_3^-} = 0$$
Urine pH = 5.8
Titratable acid = 26 mmol/day
Urine NH_4^+ = 48 mmol/day

Calculate the amount of new bicarbonate added to the blood, i.e., acid excreted.
A-64 74 mmol/day (sum of t.a. and NH_4^+, minus bicarbonate excreted).

Q-65 Which values could you predict are those for a patient with primary hyperaldosteronism?

	Urine pH	Plasma pH
a	6.9	7.55
b	8.2	7.55
c	4.8	7.30

A-65   *a*. This patient secretes excessive amounts of aldosterone, which induces potassium deficiency (because of increased renal potassium secretion). The potassium deficiency and aldosterone together then induce inappropriately large renal hydrogen-ion secretion, thereby producing a metabolic alkalosis. Note that the urine is still acid, i.e., the kidneys are not compensating for the alkalosis.

Q-66   What are the three direct effects of aldosterone on the tubule?

A-66   Increased sodium reabsorption, increased potassium secretion, and increased hydrogen-ion secretion.

Q-67   A patient has been losing large amounts of HCl because of persistent vomiting for 3 days and, therefore, has a plasma pH of 7.50. The urine pH was 8.0 at the end of day 1 and 6.9 at the end of day 3. Explain.

A-67   The alkaline urine on day 1 is the appropriate renal compensation for vomiting-induced alkalosis. The slightly acid urine on day 3 signifies that the kidneys are no longer compensating for alkalosis. This happens mainly because the progressive development of severe extracellular-volume contraction and chloride depletion stimulates hydrogen-ion secretion, preventing loss of bicarbonate in the urine. (Potassium depletion and increased aldosterone may also contribute.)

Q-68   Match each item in the top (lettered) column with appropriate item in the bottom (numbered) column ("increased" or "decreased" is used with reference to normal).
   a   Diabetic ketoacidosis
   b   Hypoventilation
   c   Excessive ingestion of sodium bicarbonate
   1   Increased plasma pH, increased plasma bicarbonate, alkaline urine
   2   Decreased plasma pH, decreased plasma bicarbonate, acidic urine
   3   Decreased plasma pH, increased plasma bicarbonate, acidic urine

A-68   a. 2
   b. 3
   c. 1

Q-69   Which of the following would you expect to find in a patient suffering from primary hypersecretion of parathyroid hormone?
   a   Increased plasma calcium
   b   Decreased plasma phosphate
   c   Increased urine calcium
   d   Increased tubular reabsorption of calcium
   e   Increased urine phosphate
   f   Increased plasma calcitonin
   g   Increased plasma 1,25-$(OH)_2D_3$

A-69   All are correct; *c* and *d* are not mutually exclusive because of the marked increase in filtered calcium. Calcitonin is reflexly increased by the increased plasma calcium. Formation of 1,25-$(OH)_2D_3$ is enhanced by parathyroid hormone.

Q-70   Which of the following would you expect to find in a person whose kidneys could not synthesize 1,25-$(OH)_2D_3$?
   a   Decreased gastrointestinal absorption of calcium

    b Decreased gastrointestinal absorption of phosphate
    c Decreased plasma calcium concentration
    d Increased plasma parathyroid-hormone concentration

A-70 All. The increased parathyroid-hormone secretion is stimulated by the low plasma calcium.

Q-71 Complete inhibition of active sodium reabsorption would cause an increase in the excretion of which of the following substances?

    a Water
    b Urea
    c Chloride
    d Glucose
    e Amino acids
    f Bicarbonate
    g Calcium

A-71 All. The reasons are all given in relevant sections of the text.

Table 1 Summary of Reabsorption and Secretion by Major Tubular Segments

	Proximal tubule R	Proximal tubule S	Henle's loop R	Henle's loop S	Distal convoluted tubule R	Distal convoluted tubule S	Collecting-duct system R	Collecting-duct system S
Organic nutrients	X							
Urea	X			(X)*			X	
Proteins, peptides	X							
Phosphate	X							
Sulfate	X							
Organic anions		X (can also be reabsorbed and/or secreted passively along tubule)						
Organic cations		X (can also be reabsorbed and/or secreted passively along tubule)						
Urate	X	X						
Sodium	X		X		X		X	
Chloride	X		X		X		X	
Water	X		X				X	
Potassium	X		X	(X)†		X	X	X
Hydrogen ions		X	X			X		X
Bicarbonate	X		X		X		X	X
Ammonium		X	(X)‡					(X)‡
Calcium	X		X		X		X	

R = reabsorption; S = secretion

*Described in note 4, Chapter 5.

†Described in note 3, Chapter 8.

‡Described in note 11, Chapter 9.

Table 2   Major Functions of the Various Collecting-Duct Cells[*]

Principal Cells
  1 Reabsorb sodium (stimulated by aldosterone)
  2 Secrete potassium (stimulated by aldosterone)
  3 Reabsorb water (stimulated by antidiuretic hormone)
Comment: Processes (1) and (2) are linked by a basolateral-membrane
  Na,K-ATPase

Type-A Intercalated Cells
  1 Secrete hydrogen ions, which effect reabsorption of bicarbonate and/or
    excretion of titratable acid (stimulated by increased P_{CO_2} and decreased
    extracellular pH)
  2 Reabsorb potassium
Comment: These two processes are linked by a luminal-membrane H,K-ATPase

Type-B Intercalated Cells
  1 Reabsorb chloride (? stimulated by chloride depletion)
  2 Secrete bicarbonate (stimulated by increased extracellular pH)
Comment: These two processes are linked by a luminal-membrane Cl/bicarbonate
  countertransporter.

---

[*]Functions of the inner medullary collecting-duct cells are not presented.

Only the most important physiological regulators are given in this table.

CLASSES
OF DIURETICS

Class	Mechanism	Major site affected
Carbonic anhydrase inhibitors	Inhibit secretion of hydrogen ions, which causes less reabsorption of bicarbonate and sodium	Proximal tubule
Loop diuretics	Inhibit Na, K, 2Cl cotransporter in luminal membrane	Thick ascending limb of Henle's loop
Thiazides	Inhibit Na, Cl cotransporter in luminal membrane	Distal convoluted tubule
Potassium-sparing diuretics*	Inhibit action of aldosterone	Cortical collecting duct
	Block sodium channels in luminal membrane	Collecting-duct system

*Except for this category, diuretics increase potassium excretion as well as sodium excretion (see text for discussion of the reasons for this increase). Aldosterone antagonists do not increase potassium excretion because they inhibit aldosterone's stimulation of potassium secretion. The sodium channel blockers also inhibit potassium secretion, in this case by reducing the amount of sodium entering the collecting duct cell for transport across the basolateral membrane by the Na,K-ATPase pumps; this reduces the activity of the pumps and, hence, the active transport of potassium into the cell.

COMPREHENSIVE MULTI-VOLUME REFERENCE WORKS

These works offer recent excellent detailed reviews of the literature in virtually every area of renal physiology and, in many cases, pathophysiology. The chapters are all written by experts in the specific areas and provide extensive lists of primary references. Many chapters in them will be cited below; for convenience, the references will not repeat the full citations of the books, which are given here, but only the information about the specific chapter being cited and the editor's name(s) to identify the book (e.g., Dennis VW: Phosphate homeostasis. In Windhager: Volume 2, Chapter 37).

Brenner BM, Rector FC Jr, eds: *The Kidney.* 4th ed. Philadelphia: WB Saunders Co; 1991.

Seldin DW, Giebisch G, eds: *The Kidney: Physiology and Pathophysiology.* 2nd ed. New York: Raven Press; 1992.

Windhager EE, ed: *Renal Physiology.* In: *Handbook of Physiology.* Section 8. New York: Oxford University Press (for the American Physiological Society); 1992.

RESEARCH TECHNIQUES
(see also Chapter 3 for clearance techniques)

Burg M: Introduction: background and development of microperfusion technique. *Kidney Int* 1982;22:417.

Handler JS, Burg MB: Application of tissue culture techniques to study of renal tubular epithelia. In Windhager: Volume 1, Chapter 10.

Kinne R: Renal plasma membranes: isolation, general properties, and biochemical components. In Windhager: Volume 2, Chapter 45.

Morel F: Methods in kidney physiology: past, present, and future. *Annu Rev Physiol* 1992;54:1.

Palmer L: Patch-clamp technique in renal physiology. *Am J Physiol* 1986;250:F379.

Symposium on methods in renal research. *Kidney Int* 1986;30:141.

Velazquez H, Wright FS: Renal micropuncture techniques. In Windhager: Volume 1, Chapter 6.

ANALYSIS OF INDIVIDUAL NEPHRON SEGMENTS

Chapters 5 to 10 concern the renal handling of specific substances. Another organizational approach to renal physiology is to look at a particular nephron segment and describe the various transport characteristics of that segment. The Suggested Readings in this section follow this latter approach.

Guder WG, Morel F: Biochemical characterization of individual nephron segments. In Windhager: Volume 2, Chapter 46.

Hebert SC: Nephron heterogeneity. In Windhager: Volume 1, Chapter 20.

Kinne RKH: Selectivity and direction: plasma membranes in renal transport. *Am J Physiol* 1991;260:F153.

Kinne RKH: Renal plasma membranes: isolation, general properties, and biochemical components. In Windhager: Volume 2, Chapter 45.

Morel F, Doucet A: Functional segmentation of the nephron. In Seldin and Giebisch: Volume 1, Chapter 31.

Sands JM, Kokko JP, Jacobson, HR: Intrarenal heterogeneity: vascular and tubular. In Seldin and Giebisch: Volume 1, Chapter 32.

CHAPTER 1

Androgue HJ: Glucose homeostasis and the kidney. *Kidney Int* 1992;42:1266.

Badr KM, Jacobson HR: Arachidonic acid metabolites and the kidney. In Brenner and Rector, Volume 1, Chapter 14.

Baker KM, Booz GW, Dostal DE: Cardiac actions of angiotensin II: role of an intra-cardiac renin-angiotensin system. *Annu Rev Physiol* 1992;54:227.

Beeuwkes R III: The vascular organization of the kidney. *Annu Rev Physiol* 1980; 42:531.

Bonvalet J-P, Pradelles P, Farman N: Segmental synthesis and actions of prostaglandins along the nephron. *Am J Physiol* 1987;253:F377.

Conrad KP, Dunn MJ: Renal prostaglandins and other eicosanoids. In Windhager: Volume 2, Chapter 35.

Daniel T: Peptide growth factors and the kidney. In Seldin and Giebisch: Volume 3, Chapter 93.

Dzau VJ, Burt DW, Pratt RE: Molecular biology of the renin-angiotensin system. *Am J Physiol* 1988;255:F563.

Fisher JW: Regulation of erythropoietin production. In Windhager: Volume 2, Chapter 51.

Ganong WF: The brain renin-angiotensin system. *Annu Rev Physiol* 1984;46:17.

Hammerman MR, O'Shea M, Miller SB: Role of growth factors in regulation of renal growth. *Annu Rev Physiol* 1993;55:305.

Kanwar YS, Venkatachalam M: Ultrastructure of glomerulus and juxtaglomerular apparatus. In Windhager: Volume 1, Chapter 1.

Kriz W, Bankir L: A standard nomenclature for structures of the kidney. *Am J Physiol* 1988;254:F1.

Kriz W, Kaissling B: Structural organization of the mammalian kidney. In Seldin and Giebisch: Volume 1, Chapter 23.

Lindpaintner K, Ganten D: The cardiac renin-angiotensin system: a synopsis of current experimental and clinical data. *NIPS* 1991;6:227.

Nord EP: Renal actions of endothelin. *Kidney Int* 1993;44:451.

Ratcliff PJ: Molecular biology of erythropoietin. *Kidney Int* 1993;44:887.

Scicli AG, Carretero OA: Renal kallikrein-kinin system. *Kidney Int* 1986;29:120.

Simonson MS, Dunn MJ: Endothelin peptides and the kidney. *Annu Rev Physiol* 1993;55:249.

Smith WL: Prostanoid biosynthesis and mechanism of action. *Am J Physiol* 1992; 263:F181.

Spivak JL, Watson AJ: Hematopoiesis and the kidney. In Seldin and Giebisch: Volume 2, Chapter 42.

Tisher CC, Madsen KM: Anatomy of the kidney. In Brenner and Rector: Volume 1, Chapter 1.

CHAPTER 2

Ballerman BJ, Zeidel ML, Gunning ME, Brenner BM: Vasoactive peptides and the kidney. In Brenner and Rector: Volume 1, Chapter 14.

Blantz RC, Thomson SC, Peterson OW, Gabbai FB: Physiologic adaptations of the tubuloglomerular feedback system. *Kidney Int* 1990;38:577.

Bonvalet J-P, Pradelles P, Farman N: Segmental synthesis and actions of prostaglandins along the nephron. *Am J Physiol* 1987;253:F377.

Campbell WB, Heinrich WL: Endothelial factors in the regulation of renin release. *Kidney Int* 1990;38:612.

Chou S-Y, Porush JG, Faubert PF: Renal medullary circulation: hormonal control. *Kidney Int* 1990;37:1.

Churchill PC: Second messengers in renin secretion. *Am J Physiol* 1985;249:F175.

Dworkin LD, Brenner BM: The renal circulations. In Brenner and Rector: Volume 1, Chapter 5.

Dworkin LD, Brenner BM: Biophysical basis of glomerular filtration. In Seldin and Giebisch: Volume 2, Chapter 29.

Heller J: Afferent and efferent glomerular arterioles: their role in glomerular filtrate formation. *NIPS* 1991;6:123.

Hura C, Stein JH: Renal blood flow. In Windhager: Volume 1, Chapter 25.

Jackson EW: Adenosine: a physiological brake on renin release. *Annu Rev Pharmacol Toxicol* 1991;31:1.

Keeton TK, Campbell WB: Control of renin release and its alteration by drugs. In: *Cardiovascular Pharmacology*. 2nd ed. New York: Raven Press; 1984:65-118.

Kopp UC, DiBona GF: The neural control of renal function. In Seldin and Giebisch: Volume 1, Chapter 33.

Maddox DA, Brenner BM: Glomerular ultrafiltration. In Brenner and Rector: Volume 1, Chapter 6.

Maddox DA, Deen WM, Brenner BM: Glomerular filtration. In Windhager: Volume 1, Chapter 13.

Mene P, Dunn MJ: Vascular, glomerular, and tubular effects of angiotensin II, kinins, and prostaglandins. In Seldin and Giebisch: Volume 1, Chapter 34.

Moss NG, Colindres RE, Gottschalk CW: Neural control of renal function. In Windhager: Volume 1, Chapter 24.

Navar LG: Physiological role of the intrarenal renin-angiotensin system (a symposium). *Fed Proc* 1986;45:1411.

Nord EP: Renal actions of endothelin. *Kidney Int* 1993;44:451.

Pallone TL, Robertson CR, Jamison RL: Renal medullary circulation. *Physiol Rev* 1990;70:885.

Schnermann JS, Briggs JP: Function of the juxtaglomerular apparatus: control of glomerular hemodynamics and renin secretion. In Seldin and Giebisch: Volume 1, Chapter 35.

Schreiner GF, Kohan DE: Regulation of renal transport processes and hemodynamics by macrophages and lymphocytes. *Am J Physiol* 1990;258:F761.

Scicli AG, Carretero OA: Renal kallikrein-kinin system. *Kidney Int* 1986;29:120.

Simonson MS, Dunn MJ: Endothelin peptides and the kidney. *Annu Rev Physiol* 1993;55:249.

Stein JH: Regulation of the renal circulation. *Kidney Int* 1990;38:571.

Steinhausen M, Endlich K, Wiegman DL: Glomerular blood flow. *Kidney Int* 1990;38:769.

Ulfendahl HR, Wolgast M: Renal circulation and lymphatics. In Seldin and Giebisch: Volume 1, Chapter 30.

CHAPTER 3

Levey AS, Perrone RD, Madias NE: Serum creatinine and renal function. *Annu Rev Physiol* 1988;39:465.

Levinsky NG, Lieberthal W: Clearance techniques. In Windhager: Volume 1, Chapter 5.

Maack T: Renal clearance and isolated kidney perfusion techniques. *Kidney Int* 1986;30:142.

Schuster VL, Seldin DW: Renal clearance. In Seldin and Giebisch: Volume 1, Chapter 28.

CHAPTER 4

Benos DJ, Sorscher EJ: Transport proteins: ion channels. In Seldin and Giebisch: Volume 1, Chapter 20.

Burckhardt G, Greger R: Principles of electrolyte transport across plasma membranes of renal tubular cells. In Windhager: Volume 1, Chapter 14.

Burckhardt G, Kinne RKH: Transport proteins: cotransporters and countertransporters. In Seldin and Giebisch: Volume 1, Chapter 19.

Geck P, Heinz E: Secondary active transport: introductory remarks. *Kidney Int* 1989;36:334-341.

Giebisch G, Boulpaep E, eds: Symposium on cotransport mechanisms in renal tubules. *Kidney Int* 1989;36:333.

Kristensen P, Ussing HH: Epithelial organization. In Seldin and Giebisch: Volume 1, Chapter 10.

Palmer LG: Renal ion channels. In Windhager: Volume 1, Chapter 16.

Palmer LG, Sackin H: Electrophysiological analysis of transepithelial transport. In Seldin and Giebisch: Volume 1, Chapter 14.

CHAPTER 5

Berry CA, Rector FC Jr: Renal transport of glucose, amino acids, sodium, chloride, and water. In Brenner and Rector: Volume 1, Chapter 7.

Deeten P, Baeyer H, Drexel H: Renal glucose transport. In Seldin and Giebisch: Volume 3, Chapter 82.

Ganapathy V, Leibach FH: Carrier-mediated reabsorption of small peptides in renal proximal tubule. *Am J Physiol* 1986;251:F945.

Grantham JJ, Chonko AM: Renal handling of organic anions and cations: excretion of uric acid. In Brenner and Rector: Volume 1, Chapter 13.

Guggino WB, Guggino SE: Renal anion transport. *Kidney Int* 1989;36:385.

Knepper MA, Roch-Ramel F: Pathways of urea transport in the mammalian kidney. *Kidney Int* 1987;31:629.

Knepper MA, Star RA: The vasopressin-regulated urea transporter in renal inner medullary collecting duct. *Am J Physiol* 1990;259:F393.

Maack T: Renal handling of proteins and polypeptides. In Windhager: Volume 2, Chapter 44.

Maack T, Park CH, Camargo MJF: Renal filtration, transport, and metabolism of proteins. In Seldin and Giebisch: Volume 3, Chapter 88.

Marsh DJ, Knepper MA: Renal handling of urea. In Windhager: Volume 2, Chapter 29.

Pritchard JB, Miller DS: Proximal tubular transport of organic anions and cations. In Seldin and Giebisch: Volume 3, Chapter 84.

Roch-Ramel F, Besseghir K, Murer H: Renal excretion and tubular transport of organic anions and cations. In Windhager: Volume 2, Chapter 48.

Saktor B: Sodium-coupled hexose transport. *Kidney Int* 1989;36:342.

Silbernagl S: Amino acids and oligopeptides. In Seldin and Giebisch: Volume 3, Chapter 83.

Silbernagl S: Tubular transport of amino acids and small peptides. In Windhager: Volume 2, Chapter 41.

Silverman M, Turner RJ: Glucose transport in the renal proximal tubule. In Windhager: Volume 2, Chapter 43.

Wortman RL: Uric acid and gout. In Seldin and Giebisch: Volume 3, Chapter 86.

Zelikovic I, Chesney RW: Sodium-coupled amino acid transport in renal tubule. *Kidney Int* 1989;36:351.

CHAPTER 6

Agre P, et al: Aquaporin CHIP: the archetypal molecular water channel. *Am J Physiol* 1993;265:F463.

Aronson PS: The renal proximal tubule: a model for diversity of anion exchangers and stilbene-sensitive anion transporters. *Annu Rev Physiol* 1989;51:419.

Berry CA, Rector FC Jr: Renal transport of glucose, amino acids, sodium, chloride, and water. In Brenner and Rector: Volume 1, Chapter 7.

Breyer MD, Jacobson HR, Hebert RL: Cellular mechanisms of prostaglandin E_2 and vasopressin interactions in the collecting duct. *Kidney Int* 1990;38:618.

Culpepper RM: $Na^+=K^+=2Cl^-$ cotransport in the thick ascending limb of Henle. *Hospital Practice* June 15, 1989:217-242.

Dubinsky WP Jr: The physiology of epithelial chloride channels. *Hospital Practice* Jan. 15, 1989:69-80.

Greger R: Chloride transport in thick ascending limb, distal convolution, and collecting duct. *Annu Rev Physiol* 1988;50:111.

Jamison RL, Gehrig JJ Jr: Urinary concentration and dilution: physiology. In Windhager: Volume 2, Chapter 27.

Kinter LB, Huffman WF, Stassen FL: Antagonists of the antidiuretic activity of vaso-pressin. *Am J Physiol* 1988;254:F165.

Kirk KL, Schafer JA: Water transport and osmoregulation by antidiuretic hormone in terminal nephron segments. In Seldin and Giebisch: Volume 2, Chapter 46.

Knepper MA, Rector FC Jr: Urinary concentration and dilution. In Brenner and Rector: Volume 1, Chapter 9.

Koeppen BM, Stanton BA: Sodium chloride transport: distal nephron. In Seldin and Giebisch: Volume 2, Chapter 55.

Kokko JP, Baum M: Chloride transport. In Windhager: Volume 1, Chapter 17.

Maron S, Winaver J, Dagan D: Single-channel techniques applied to kidney proximal tubule apical membranes. *NIPS* 1990;5:194.

Palmer LG: Epithelial Na channels: function and diversity. *Annu Rev Physiol* 1992;54:51.

Reeves WB, Andreoli TE: Renal epithelial chloride channels. *Annu Rev Physiol* 1992;54:29.

Reeves WB, Andreoli TE: Sodium chloride transport in the loop of Henle. In Seldin and Giebisch: Volume 2, Chapter 54.

Roy DR, Layton HE, Jamison RL: Countercurrent mechanism and its regulation. In Seldin and Giebisch: Volume 2, Chapter 45.

Sasaki S, Marumo F: Mechanisms of transcellular chloride transport in mammalian renal proximal tubules. *NIPS* 1989;4:18.

Schafer JA: Transepithelial osmolarity differences, hydraulic conductivities, and vol-ume absorption in the proximal tubule. *Annu Rev Physiol* 1990;52:709.

Schafer JA, Reeves WB, Andreoli TE: Mechanisms of fluid transport across renal tubules. In Windhager: Volume 1, Chapter 15.

Schreiner GF, Kohan DE: Regulation of renal transport processes and hemodynamics by macrophages and lymphocytes. *Am J Physiol* 1990;258:F761.

Skorechi KL, Brown D, Ercolani L, Ausiello DA: Molecular mechanisms of vaso-pressin action in the kidney. In Windhager: Volume 2, Chapter 26.

Smith PR, Benos DJ: Epithelial Na channels. *Annu Rev Physiol* 1991;53:509.

Stephenson JL: Urinary concentration and dilution: models. In Windhager: Volume 2, Chapter 30.

Stokes, JB: Electroneutral NaCl transport in the distal tubule. *Kidney Int* 1989;36:427.

Verkman AS: Water channels in cell membranes. *Annu Rev Physiol* 1992;54:97.

Weinstein AM: Sodium chloride transport: proximal nephron. In Seldin and Giebisch: Volume 2, Chapter 53.

See also articles under "Analysis of Individual Nephron Segments."

CHAPTER 7

Atlas SA, Maack T: Atrial natriuretic factor. In Windhager: Volume 2, Chapter 33.

Ballerman BJ, Zeide ML: Atrial natriuretic hormone. In Seldin and Giebisch: Volume 2, Chapter 51.

Bastl CP, Hayslett JP: The cellular action of aldosterone in target epithelia. *Kidney Int* 1992;42:250.

Bertorello AM, Katz AI: Short-term regulation of renal Na-K-ATPase activity: physi-ological relevance and cellular mechanisms. *Am J Physiol* 1993;265:F743.

Brenner BM, Ballerman BJ, Gunning ME, Zeidel ML: Diverse biological actions of atrial natriuretic peptide. *Physiol Rev* 1990;70:665.

Breyer MD: Regulation of water and salt transport in collecting duct through calcium-dependent signaling mechanisms. *Am J Physiol* 1991;260:F1.

Cogan MG: Renal effects of atrial natriuretic factor. *Annu Rev Physiol* 1990;52:699.

Dzau VJ: Renal and circulatory mechanisms in congestive heart failure. *Kidney Int* 1987;31:1402.

Fitzsimmons JT: Physiology and pathophysiology of thirst and sodium appetite. In Seldin and Giebisch: Volume 2, Chapter 44.

Funder JW: Aldosterone actions. *Annu Rev Physiol* 1993;55:115.

Garg LC: Actions of adrenergic and cholinergic drugs on renal tubular cells. *Pharmacol Rev* 1992;44:81.

Gellai M: Modulation of vasopressin antidiuretic action by renal alpha$_2$-adrenoceptors. *Am J Physiol* 1990;259:F1.

Goetz KL: Renal natriuretic peptide (urdilatin?) and atriopeptin: evolving concepts. *Am J Physiol* 1991;261:F921.

Gonzalez-Campoy JM, Knox FJ: Integrated responses of the kidney to alterations in extracellular fluid volume. In Seldin and Giebisch: Volume 2, Chapter 56.

Hall JE, Brands MW: The renin-angiotensin-aldosterone systems: renal mechanisms and circulatory homeostasis. In Seldin and Giebisch: Volume 2, Chapter 40.

Hamlyn JM, Ludens JH: Nonatrial natriuretic hormones: In Seldin and Giebisch: Volume 2, Chapter 52.

Ichikawa I, Harris RC: Angiotensin actions in the kidney: renewed insight into the old hormone. *Kidney Int* 1991;40:583.

Inagami T, Harris RC: Molecular insights into angiotensin II receptor subtypes. *NIPS* 1993;8:215.

Knox FG, Granger JP: Control of sodium excretion: an integrative approach. In Windhager: Volume 1, Chapter 21.

Kopp UC, DiBona GF: The neural control of renal function. In Seldin and Giebisch: Volume 1, Chapter 33.

Laragh JH: The renin system and the renal regulation of blood pressure. In Seldin and Giebisch: Volume 2, Chapter 39.

Maack TM: Receptors of atrial natriuretic factor. *Annu Rev Physiol* 1992;54:11.

Moss NG, Colindres RE, Gottschalk CW: Neural control of renal function. In Windhager: Volume 1, Chapter 24.

Oparil S, Wyss JM: Atrial natriuretic factor in central cardiovascular control. *NIPS* 1993;8:223.

Peterson TV, Benjamin BA: The heart and control of renal excretion: neural and endocrine mechanisms. *FASEB J* 1992;6:2923.

Quinn SJ: Regulation of aldosterone secretion. *Annu Rev Physiol* 1988;50:409.

Robertson GL: Regulation of vasopressin secretion. In Seldin and Giebisch: Volume 2, Chapter 43.

Ruskaoho H, Vuolteenaho O: Regulation of atrial natriuretic peptide secretion. *NIPS* 1993;8:261.

Schafer JA, Hawk CT: Regulation of sodium channels in the cortical collecting duct by AVP and mineralocorticoids. *Kidney Int* 1992;41:255.

Schneider EG: In water deprivation, osmolarity becomes an important determinant of aldosterone secretion. *NIPS* 1990;5:197.

Selden DW, Giebisch G: *The Regulation of Sodium and Chloride Balance.* New York: Raven Press; 1989.

Stokes JB: Sodium and potassium transport by the collecting duct. *Kidney Int* 1990;38:679.

Wilcox CS, Baylis C, Wingo CS: Glomerular-tubular balance and proximal regulation. In Seldin and Giebisch: Volume 2, Chapter 50.

Zeeuw DJ, Janssen WMT, deJong PE: Atrial natriuretic factor: its (patho)physiological significance in humans. *Kidney Int* 1992;41:1115.

Zeidel ML: Renal actions of atrial natriuretic peptide: regulation of collecting duct sodium and water transport. *Annu Rev Physiol* 1990;52:747.

CHAPTER 8

Androgue HJ, Madias NE: Changes in plasma potassium concentration during acute acid-base disturbances. *Am J Med* 1981;71:456.

Giebisch G, Malnic G, Berliner RW: Renal transport and control of potassium excretion. In Brenner and Rector: Volume 1, Chapter 8.

Rabinowitz L: Do splanchnic potassium receptors initiate a kaliuretic reflex? *NIPS* 1991;6:166.

Rosa RM, Williams ME, Epstein FH: Extrarenal potassium metabolism. In Seldin and Giebisch: Volume 2, Chapter 59.

Seldin DW, ed: *The Regulation of Potassium Balance*. New York: Raven Press; 1988.

Stanton BA, Giebisch G: Renal potassium transport. In Windhager: Volume 1. Chapter 19.

Stokes JB: Sodium and potassium transport by the collecting duct. *Kidney Int* 1990;38:679.

Warnock, DG, Eveloff J: K-Cl cotransport systems. *Kidney Int* 1989;36:412.

Wingo CS, Cain BD: The renal H-K-ATPase: physiological significance and role in potassium homeostasis. *Annu Rev Physiol* 1993;55:323.

Wright FS, Giebisch G: Regulation of potassium excretion. In Seldin and Giebisch: Volume 2, Chapter 59.

Young DB: Quantitative analysis of aldosterone's role in potassium regulation. *Am J Physiol* 1988;255:F811.

See also articles listed under "Analysis of Individual Nephron Segments."

CHAPTER 9

Alpern RJ: Cell mechanisms of proximal tubule acidification. *Physiol Rev* 1990;70:79.

Alpern RJ, Rector FC Jr: Renal acidification: cellular mechanisms of tubular transport and regulation. In Windhager: Volume 1, Chapter 18.

Alpern RJ, Stone DK, Rector FC Jr: Renal acidification mechanisms. In Brenner and Rector, Volume 1, Chapter 9.

Boron WF, Boulpaep EL: The electrogenic Na/HCO_3 cotransporter. *Kidney Int* 1989;36:392.

Cogan MG, Quan AH: Renal acidification: integrated tubular responses. In Windhager: Volume 1, Chapter 22.

DuBose TD Jr: Kinetics of CO_2 exchange in the kidney. *Annu Rev Physiol* 1988;50:653.

DuBose TD Jr: Reclamation of filtered bicarbonate. *Kidney Int* 1990;38:584.

Galla JH, Gifford JD, Luke RG, Rome L: Adaptations to chloride-depletion alkalosis. *Am J Physiol* 1991;261:R771.

Garg LC: Respective roles of H-ATPase and H-K-ATPase in ion transport in the kidney. *J Am Soc Nephrol* 1991;2:949.

Gennari FJ, Maddox DA: Renal regulation of acid-base homeostasis: integrated response. In Seldin and Giebisch: Volume 2, Chapter 78.

Gluck SL: Cellular and molecular aspects of renal H^+ transport. *Hospital Practice* May 15, 1989:149-166.

Halperin ML, Kamel KS, Ethier JH, Stinebaugh BJ, Jungas RL: Biochemistry and physiology of ammonium excretion. In Seldin and Giebisch: Volume 2, Chapter 76.

Hamm LL, Alpern RJ: Cellular mechanisms of renal tubular acidification. In Seldin and Giebisch: Volume 2, Chapter 74.

Kill F: The paradox of renal bicarbonate reabsorption. *NIPS* 1990;5:13.

Knepper MA, Packer R, Good DW: Ammonium transport in the kidney. *Physiol Rev* 1989;69:179.

Kurtzman NA: Disorders of distal acidification. *Kidney Int* 1990;38:720.

Moe OW, Preisig PA, Alpern RJ: Cellular model of proximal tubule NaCl and Na-HCO_3 absorption. *Kidney Int* 1990;38:605.

Preisig PA, Alpern RJ: Basolateral membrane H/HCO_3 transport in renal tubules. *Kidney Int* 1991;39:1077.

Schuster VL: Function and regulation of collecting duct intercalated cells. *Annu Rev Physiol* 1993;55:267.

Seldin DW, Giebisch G, eds: *The Regulation of Acid-Base Balance*. New York: Raven Press; 1990.

Steinmetz PR: Cellular organization of urinary acidification. *Am J Physiol* 1986;251:F173.

Tannen RL: Renal ammonia production and excretion. In Windhager: Volume 1, Chapter 23.

Walser M: Roles of urea production, ammonium excretion, and amino acid oxidation in acid-base balance. *Am J Physiol* 1986;250:F181.

Weinman EJ: Regulation of the renal brush border membrane Na-H exchanger. *Annu Rev Physiol* 1993;55:289.

See also articles listed under "Analysis of Individual Nephron Segments."

CHAPTER 10

Austin LA, Heath H III: Calcitonin: physiology and pathophysiology. *N Engl J Med* 1981;304:269.

Berndt TJ, Knox FG: Renal regulation of phosphate excretion. In Seldin and Giebisch: Volume 2, Chapter 71.

Brown AJ, Dusso AS, Slatopolsky E: Vitamin D. In Seldin and Giebisch: Volume 2, Chapter 41.

Bronner F: Renal calcium transport: mechanisms and regulation—an overview. *Am J Physiol* 1989;257:F707.

Carafoli E: The calcium pumping ATPase of the plasma membrane. *Annu Rev Physiol* 1991;53:531.

Caverzasio J, Bonjour J-P: IGF-1, a key regulator of renal phosphate transport and 1,25-dihydroxyvitamin D_3 production during growth. *NIPS* 1991;6:206.

Costanzo LS, Windhager EE: Renal regulation of calcium balance. In Seldin and Giebisch: Volume 2, Chapter 66.

Costanzo LS, Windhager EE: Renal tubular transport of calcium. In Windhager: Volume 2, Chapter 36.

Dennis VW: Phosphate homeostasis. In Windhager: Volume 2, Chapter 37.

Friedman PA, Gesek FA: Calcium transport in renal epithelial cells. *Am J Physiol* 1993;264:F181.

Gross M, Kumar R: Vitamin D endocrine system and calcium and phosphorus homeostasis. In Windhager: Volume 2, Chapter 38.

Muer H, Biber J: Renal tubular phosphate transport. In Seldin and Giebisch: Volume 2, Chapter 70.

Muff R, Fischer JA: Parathyroid hormone receptors in control of proximal tubule function. *Annu Rev Physiol* 1992;54:67.

Pocotte SS, Ehrenstein G, Fitzpatrick LA: Regulation of parathyroid hormone secretion. *Endocrine Rev* 1991;12:291.

Rouse D, Suki WN: Renal control of extracellular calcium. *Kidney Int* 1990;38:700.

Suki WM, Rouse D: Renal transport of calcium, magnesium, and phosphate. In Brenner and Rector: Volume 1, Chapter 10.

See also articles listed under "Analysis of Individual Nephron segments."

APPENDIX A. DIURETICS

Breyer J, Jacobson HR: Molecular mechanisms of diuretic agents. *Annu Rev Med* 1990;41:265.

Lane F, ed: Physiology of diuretic action. *Renal Physiol* 1987;10:129.

Martinez-Maldonado M, Cordova HR: Cellular and molecular aspects of the renal effects of diuretic agents. *Kidney Int* 1990;38:632.

Puschett JB, Winaver J: Effects of diuretics on renal function. In Windhager: Volume 2, Chapter 50.

Rose BD: Diuretics. *Kidney Int* 1991;39:336.

Suki WN, Eknoyan G: Physiology of diuretic action. In Windhager: Volume 3, Chapter 108.

STAYING UP-TO-DATE

The most painless way for a busy clinician not specializing in nephrology to follow important developments in renal physiology is to read the excellent reviews that appear frequently in the *New England Journal of Medicine* and *Hospital Practice*. They are usually succinct and emphasize the clinical implications of new research findings. More detailed reviews are to be found in the *Annual Review of Physiology, News in Physiological Sciences (NIPS), Endocrine Reviews, Recent Progress in Hormone Research*, and the specialty journals for renal physiology, notably the *American Journal of Physiology (Renal and Electrolyte Section), Kidney International, Renal Physiology*, and *Mineral and Electrolyte Metabolism*. The journals *Hypertension* and *Circulation Research* frequently have reviews dealing with the renin-angiotensin system. The *Annual Review of Medicine* and the *Annual Review of Pharmacology* present clinically relevant material.

INDEX

ISBN 0-07-067009-9

90000>

9 780070 670099